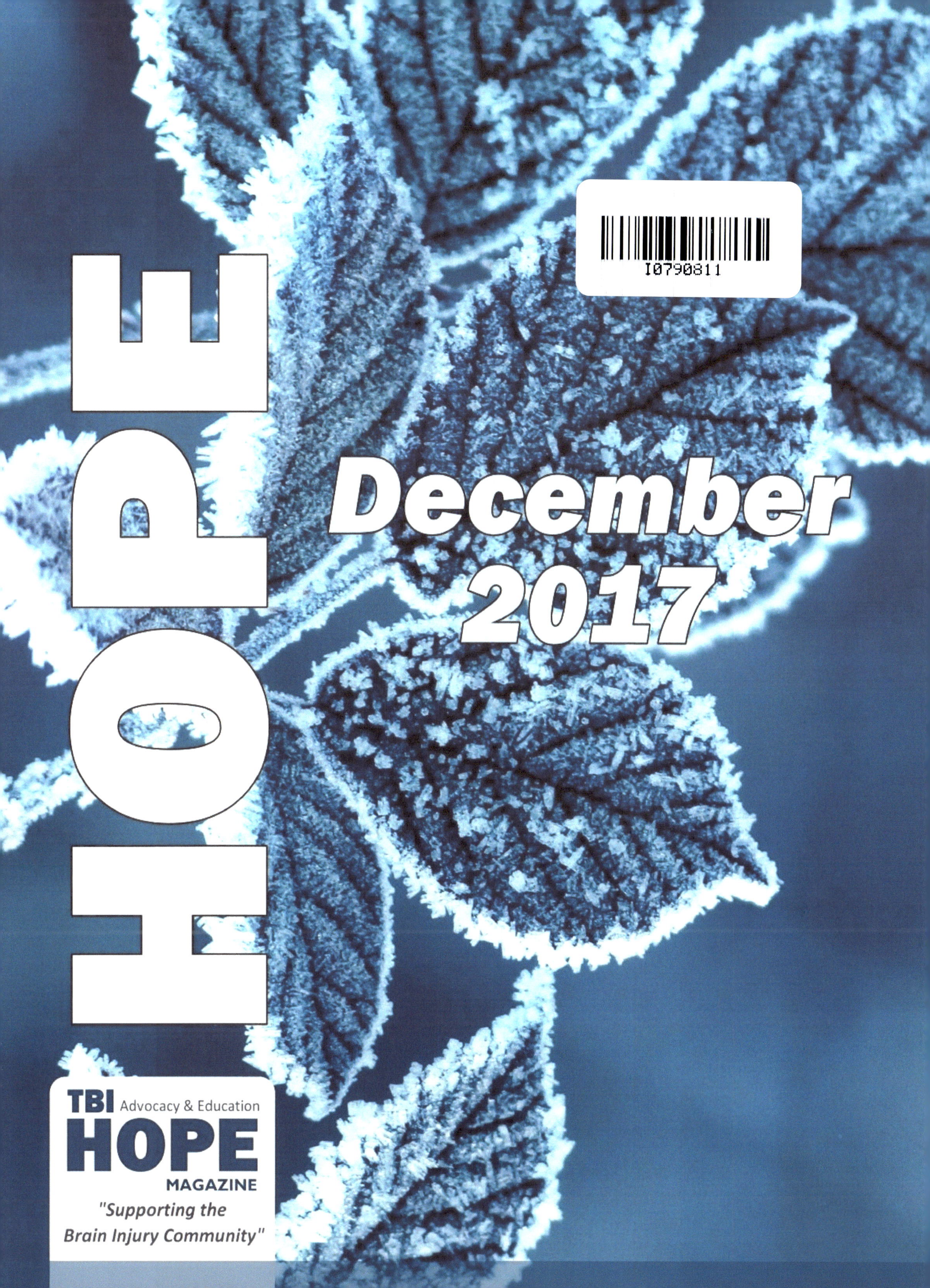

HOPE
December
2017
TBI Advocacy & Education
HOPE
MAGAZINE
"Supporting the
Brain Injury Community"

Welcome

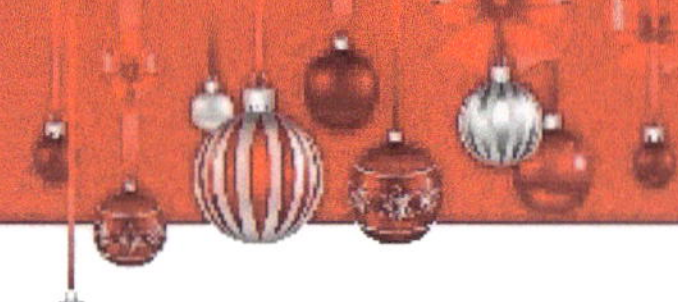

TBI HOPE MAGAZINE

Serving All Impacted by Brain Injury

December 2017

Publisher
David A. Grant

Editor
Sarah Grant

Contributing Writers
Michelle Bartlett
Nicole Bingaman
Jim Martin
Keely Parker
Rosemary Rawlins
Barbara Stahura
Mike Strand
Hilary Zayed

Amazing Cartoonist
Patrick Brigham

*FREE subscriptions at
www.TBIHopeMagazine.com*

Welcome to the December 2017 issue of TBI HOPE Magazine!

We are pleased to offer our annual holiday-themed issue to you. The holidays can be such a fun and exciting time of year for many, but living with a brain injury does change things a bit.

It's all too easy to get overwhelmed this time of year by pressures we navigated with ease in lives past. Family get-togethers are wonderful, but the chaos can overwhelm those living with a brain injury. We tire more easily, and many of us have challenges with seemingly simple tasks like following conversations in a busy room.

We can add to this the financial pressures that come with the holidays, the mainstream media feeding us endless commercials pressuring us to spend more. This in light of the fact that many are just getting by.

This holiday season, as we have done every year since my own brain injury, we are staying small. We will get together with small circles of family and friends, avoid chaos, and focus on things that are truly meaningful.

I encourage you to be good to yourself, to take it as easy as you are able to, and to rejoice in those things that are going well in your life.

Happy Holidays,

David A. Grant
Publisher

Contents

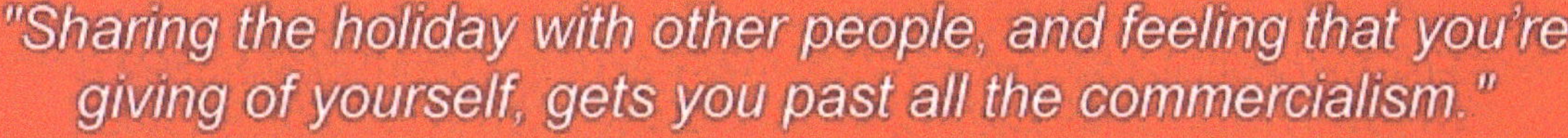

"Sharing the holiday with other people, and feeling that you're giving of yourself, gets you past all the commercialism."

~Caroline Kennedy

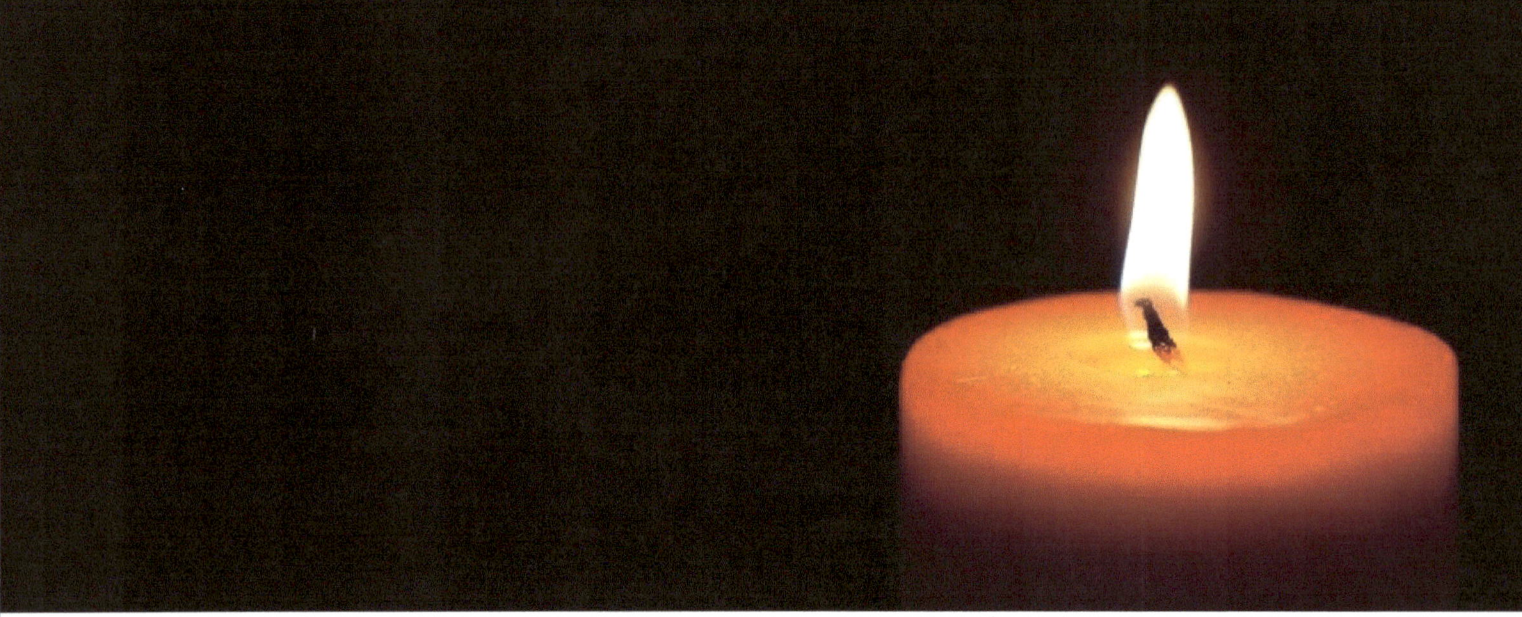

Intentions to Light the Way

By Rosemary Rawlins

The holidays are a time of rushing around, squeezing the budget, and sometimes losing our tempers as we try to cram more and more into each day. And if you're a caregiver, you may find it's difficult to schedule time off for yourself and to find gifts and meaningful ways of celebrating that will honor and delight the person in your care. For caregivers, money is often tight, making the holidays feel more dismal than other times of the year because we can't do what we wish, and can't give what we want to give.

But here's another way of looking at the holiday season. It's the turning of a corner, the dawn of a New Year. It's *supposed* to be a celebration! So instead of rushing, why not take one hour to quiet your mind? Just one hour.

> ## "Why not take one hour to quiet your mind?"

Light a candle. Take a breath.

Now close your eyes and review the year you just lived through. Watch your mental slideshow month to month, and pause at the heartening moments. Remember those who have helped you. See the faces of your friends, your partner, your children or parents.

Now open your eyes and look at the candle. Imagine the light is creating a path for you. Who do you want to be in the coming year? What can you do to make that happen? Making resolutions is common at the New Year, and breaking them is even more common. But what if, instead of a resolution, you set your intentions? This is a worthwhile tradition to start, and it doesn't cost any money at all.

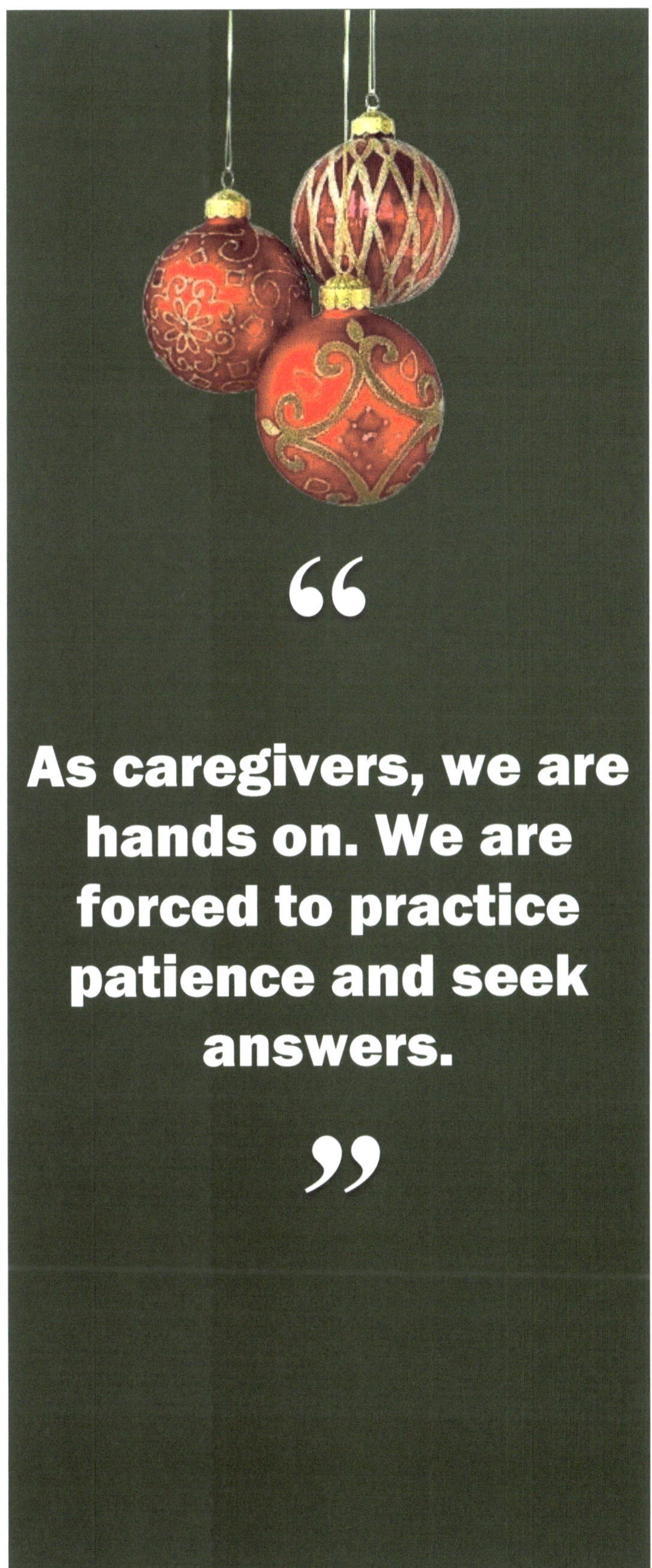

I've had some emotional ups and downs this year, and I think a lot of people are concerned about ongoing disputes that have caused divisions that seem to be growing deeper in our country and abroad. Tension in the news can create tension in families. That's why it's important to step back and make sure we are not engaging in passive aggressive ways when we disagree with family members on issues or beliefs.

As caregivers, we are hands on. We are forced to practice patience and seek answers. The people we care for depend on us to be consistent and reasonable, stable and strong, yet sometimes it's hard for us to cope amid all the turmoil around us.

Setting our intentions may be one way of realigning ourselves with our values and goals, so we can continue to give care in a positive way.

With that in mind, I'll share with you what my intentions are for 2018:

> *To listen and respond in love*
> *To have strong convictions and*
> *eloquent ways of sharing them*
> *To be mindful when communicating,*
> *without belittling*
> *To try to understand others*
> *even when I disagree with them*
> *To strive for peace in myself,*
> *my family, and my world*

This is a tall order. It's especially tall because I know I will fail repeatedly. But recognizing that I sometimes fly off the handle, or misinterpret what others are saying and take offense, or fail to listen closely is an important step in figuring out what I might do to calm myself and to be a better caregiver going forward.

I know that I'm responsible for half of the stress I feel and blame on others. I think it's a common affliction—the tendency to react rather than think through a response to what we perceive as annoyance. And so I'm going to take responsibility and try to open my mind a little bit more.

One of my favorite carols is "Let There be Peace on Earth, and Let it Begin with Me." The lyrics are heartwarming, but this year, this song leaves me disheartened because there is *so little* peace on earth.

I hope that by setting my intentions, I might be reminded more often that I need to look within as often as I look outside for the peace I seek, and try to be a part of the solution instead of simply feeling helpless.

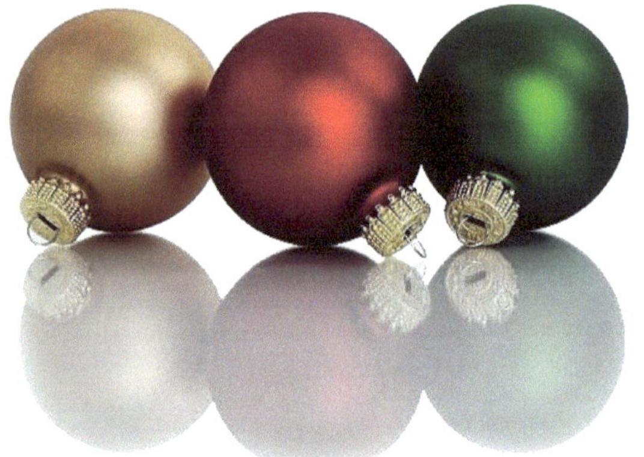

Meet Rosemary Rawlins

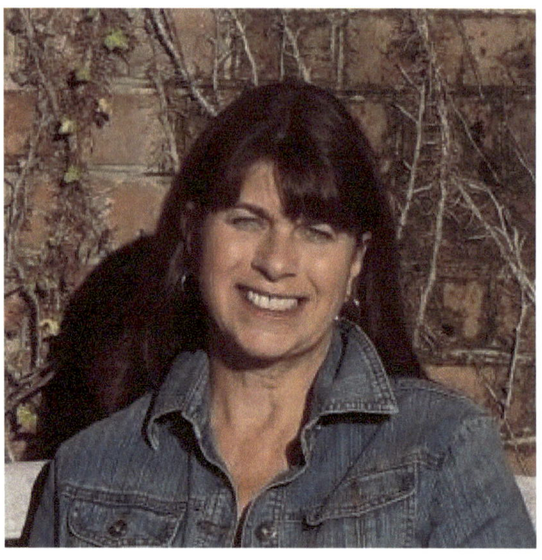

Rosemary Rawlins is the author of Learning by Accident: A Caregiver's True Story of Fear, Family, and Hope, an inspirational memoir about learning and growing through adversity.

When Rosemary's husband suffered a severe traumatic brain injury after a car hit him on his bike, she struggled for two years to bring him back home and back to himself, and when he was finally better, she fell apart. Rosemary has had many years of experience as a full-time caregiver for loved ones with brain injury, dementia, and COPD, and has a keen understanding of caregiver stress.

She is also Editor of BrainLine blogs and a national speaker on caregiving topics. You can learn more about Rosemary at: www.rosemaryrawlins.com

Great works are performed not by strength but by perseverance.

~Samuel Jackson

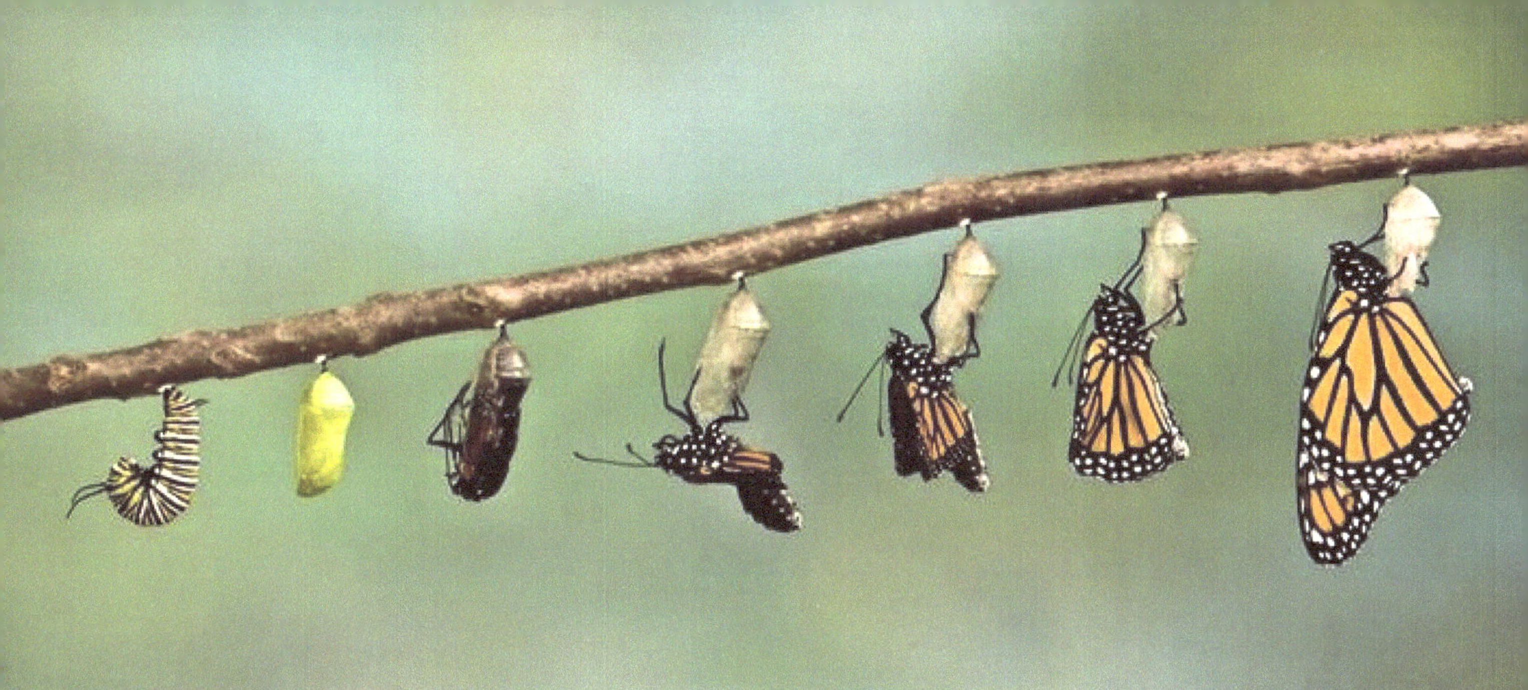

Transitions

By Jim Martin

As I continue to recover from my TBI, I have come to realize and appreciate that this has been a period of transition, rather than change, in my life. The words "change" and "transition" are not necessarily equivalent. For me, "change" suggests an event, whereas "transition" infers how I react and respond to that event. Yes, there have been events, such as the day I experienced the TBI. That, as I now understand, was a change in my life. However, the recovery from that event has no endpoint and I have needed to alter my perspective. For now, this period of time is one of transition and I do not know where it will lead. I can only hope that I will continue to be productive and helpful to others, despite the limitations afforded by my TBI and resulting memory impairment.

In understanding this process I have drawn great solace from a book entitled "The Way of Transition," by William Bridges. In it, he describes three phases of transition, and as I now understand what has occurred for me, it makes a lot of sense. First, there is the ending of my day-to-day former life, where I was a trial lawyer for thirty years. In that phase, there is recognition of the loss and the need to let go of my old reality, attitudes and, most importantly, self-image.

Addressing (or not) those issues led to feelings of sadness, isolation, fear, apathy, and anger. This was definitely not an easy process, nor did it occur quickly. Next, is a period called the neutral zone - not being my old self as a trial lawyer, and yet not being someone with a new identity and purpose. To say the least, it was, and at times, continues to

> ## "I can only hope that I will continue to be productive and helpful to others."

be a confusing time. Nothing seems real; yet, at the same time, everything seems potentially possible, just different. I am still in this neutral zone, comfortably so for the moment, but also itching to find my next pursuit. The third phase of the transition process will be when I can take hold and identify with a new outlook and a new reality of what the future may hold, in effect, a new chapter in my life.

As suggested in the book, identifying with being in transition allowed me to come to terms with change. Over time, I was able to refocus my energy on dealing with my new situation, whether I defined it as "good" or "bad," unrestrained by my attitudes/behaviors which may have been more developed for, and perhaps more appropriate for, my old situation.

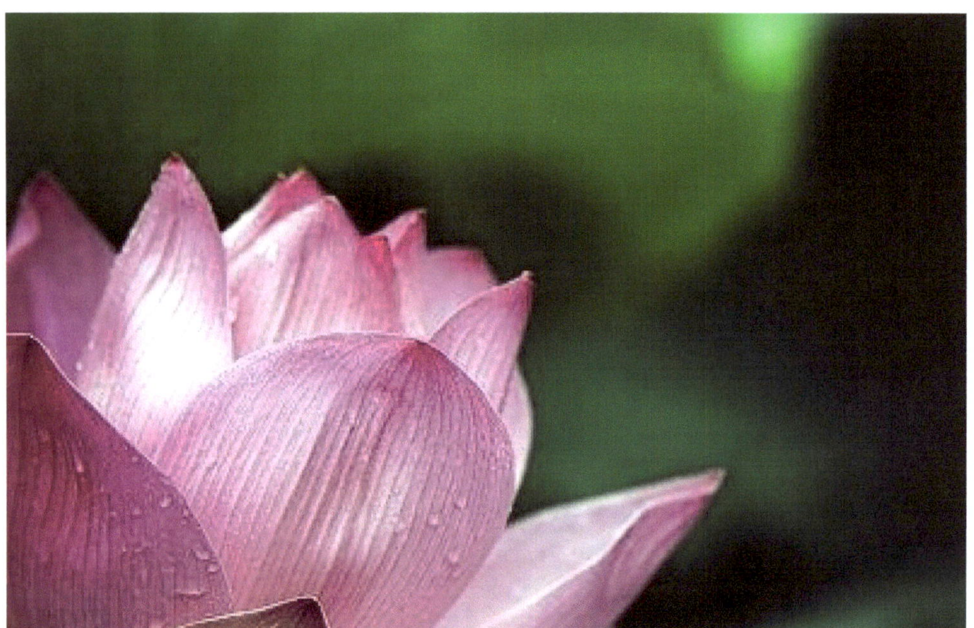

Along with the many differences which I have experienced over the past nearly seven years, it has also become apparent to me that the deficits resulting from my TBI are virtually invisible. In other words, to almost the entire world, I look and act "normal," (however that may be defined.) And the personal frustration at accepting that reality - looking normal - has, at times, been overwhelming. Fortunately, I was willing to seek the help of a few professional therapists, one of whom specializes in brain injured patients. With their patience and understanding, I've come to realize that while I may "appear" to present to others is very, very different than what I experience and, in fact, that my deficits are real. Once I was able to acknowledge that reality, I was willing to see that I was in the "neutral zone."

While I have accepted and adopted these suggestions, being in the "neutral zone" is and has been challenging, particularly as I age. Whereas the first phase is marked by an event, and hopefully the third phase will also be marked by some form of an event, the neutral zone has been like being in "no man's land," an uneventful time in my life, where I am a person with no real identity. Now, however, being able to sustain hope in the face of a dramatic difference, I find myself more willing to weather the storm. Moreover, I have hope that coming out of this period of transition will allow me to be authentic - knowing myself better, willing to express who I truly am, and having the faith and confidence to trust that who I am is real, and that I am a person capable of functioning in this world.

In many ways, I've also appreciated the difference between the words perspective and perception. Although there are adequate dictionary definitions, following my TBI, life was determined more by perception than accurate perspective. I viewed how others responded and/or treated me with a skewed perception, surely influenced by the TBI, and enhanced by my own selfishness and self-pity. It has been nearly seven years since the accident leading to my TBI, and it has only been in the past 30-36 months that my perspective has changed. For example, what my true limitations as well as assets are in reality, as compared to my perception. And, how I thought others were thinking of me and what I could or could not do, has slowly transformed. It has only occurred as the result of my willingness to accept my new, current reality, and an optimism that a new, albeit different, life lies ahead.

From my perspective, all of the gifts which I have received so far have been achieved, in substantial part, because I have been able to maintain balance. Recognizing and realizing that I am very fortunate to still be alive, and while I continue to struggle at times with emotional and physical pain, there remain so many opportunities which have and will continue to present themselves as long as I maintain a healthy perspective.

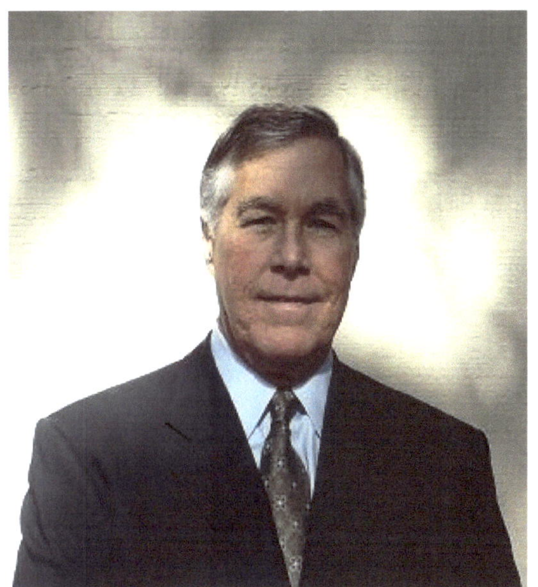

Meet Jim Martin

After 30 years practicing law as a trial attorney primarily representing physicians in medical malpractice litigation, Jim is a brain injury survivor whose career ended in December, 2010 when he experienced a significant traumatic brain injury, and resulting permanent memory impairment. Jim volunteers with the Alzheimer's Association, where he is a Board member, attends support group meetings with Brain Injury Connections NW, is a member of Brain Injury Alliance of Oregon, and volunteers at a local Portland, Oregon hospital. To stay connected with the legal community, Jim mentors newly admitted lawyers with the Oregon State Bar.

Living With Hope
By Patrick Brigham

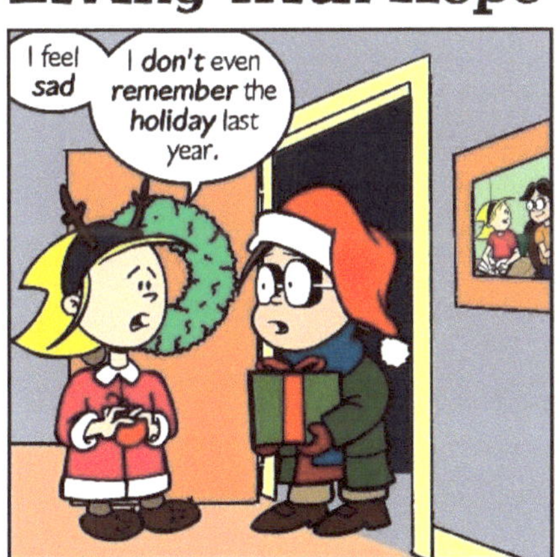

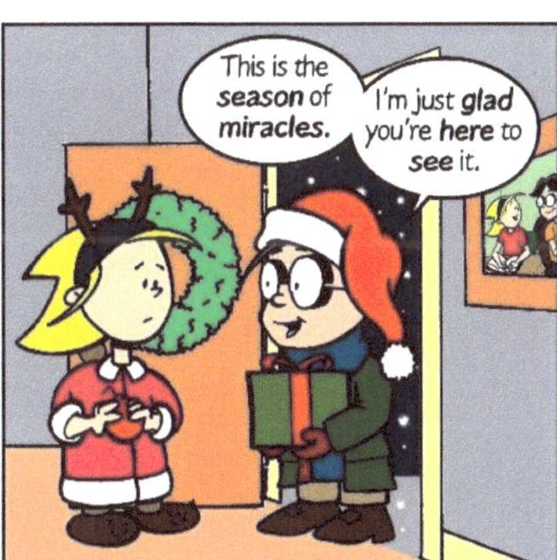

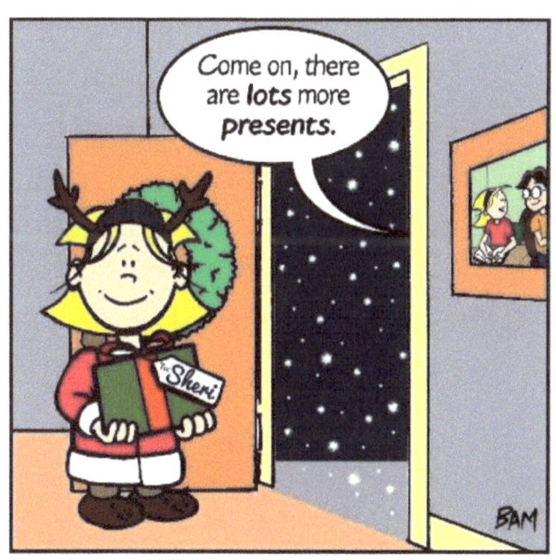

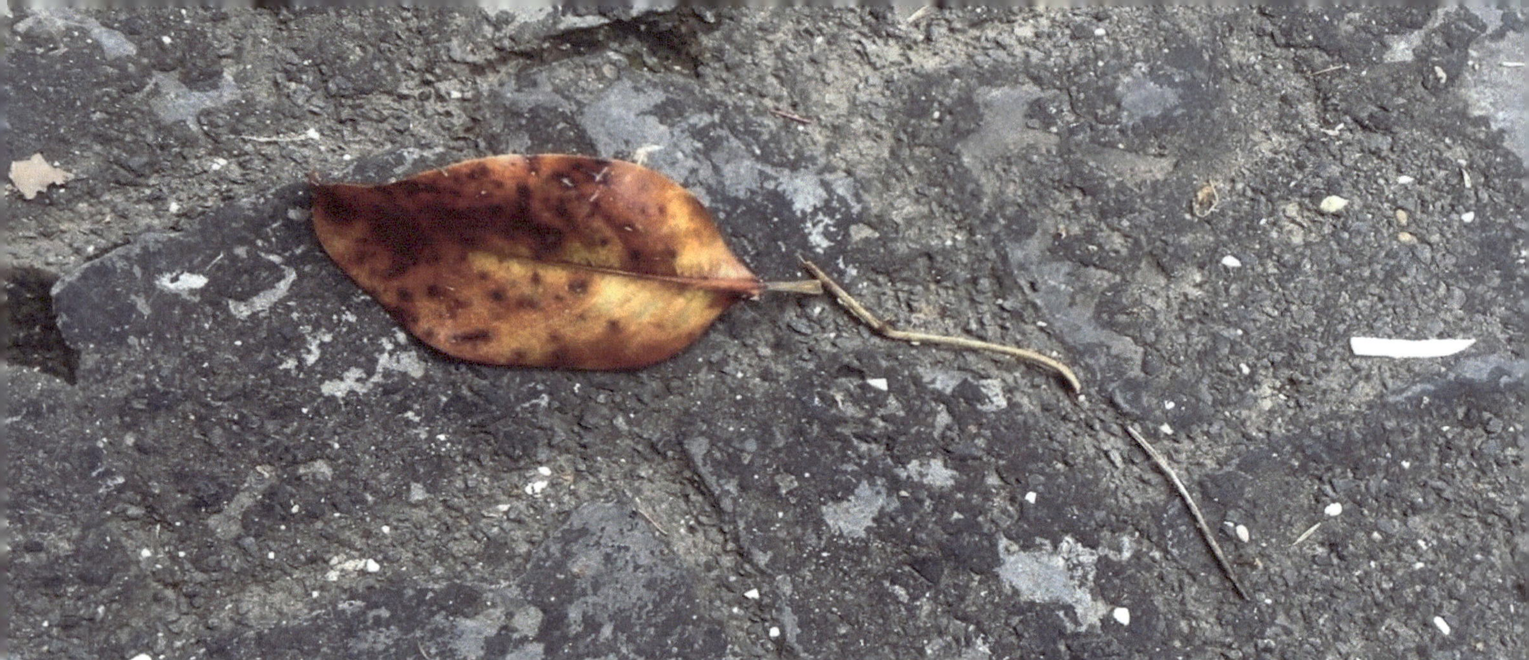

Pretty No More
By Nicole Bingaman

I wrote a poem about a year ago as I was watching the effects of my then twenty-five-year-old son's brain injury. I wondered, "What if I were the one who sustained the brain injury? How would my tribe respond?"

I thought about a couple we met during my son's first days in rehab, Paul and Tammy. They were in their forties and dating just before fate introduced us. Paul was riding his motorcycle a short distance on the local Air force base where he worked. He was retired and employed as a civilian.

Paul appeared to be one of these guys who had it all. He was attractive, had been part of a security squadron in the air force, and he was in love. In many ways Paul did have it all, until the night he got on his motorcycle, didn't put on a helmet, and a young, inexperienced driver failed to stop and collided into him.

When I met Paul, he had come out of an accident that left him kissing death's door. He was a survivor, but there was profound damage. Paul's language skills were poor at best, and he had countless other brain injury associated issues.

But Paul had a sassy, strong, powerhouse of a woman by his side, and together they would come to move mountains. What I first noticed about Tammy was that she came on strong. You knew she was in the room, and you knew she meant business, but that was the best thing for Paul. She wasn't messing around. And nothing was going to stand in her way of both helping and loving Paul.

The second thing I noticed and the thing that stuck is that Tammy adored Paul. It was about eight months after his accident when they were married, and I have been following their love story ever since. You see…it inspires me. Love doesn't have to come in a neat, pretty package to be love. We know that brain injury is messy, but these two make it look a bit magical.

Talking to Paul is a challenge. His language database is still messed up, and his laughter prevails at times over his words. I remember a conversation with him that went something like this…"Hi Paul, how are you today?" And the first words of his response were appropriate, "I'm doing fine…agweaid, gwet gonegoo whap news…" followed by hardcore laughter. Being new to the world of brain injury, I was fairly lost.

But I knew enough to know Paul's wires were crossed. He appeared to fully know what he was saying, but he could not get it out so that I could understand.

Tammy came into Paul's life before his accident, and has loved him full and well ever since.

This poem asks a series of questions, and as caregivers and survivors there are endless questions that swirl through our minds. I'd like to think of myself as the friend that sticks by no matter what, but I also know that in our humanity sometimes things just feel incredibly hard.

I wrote this poem in honor of Paul, and those like Tammy who chose to stay, despite the challenges. We really don't ever know the answers to what we will do our how we will respond, but I do know with certainty within the family of brain injury I have met some of the most loving, inspiring and gentle people I have ever witnessed.

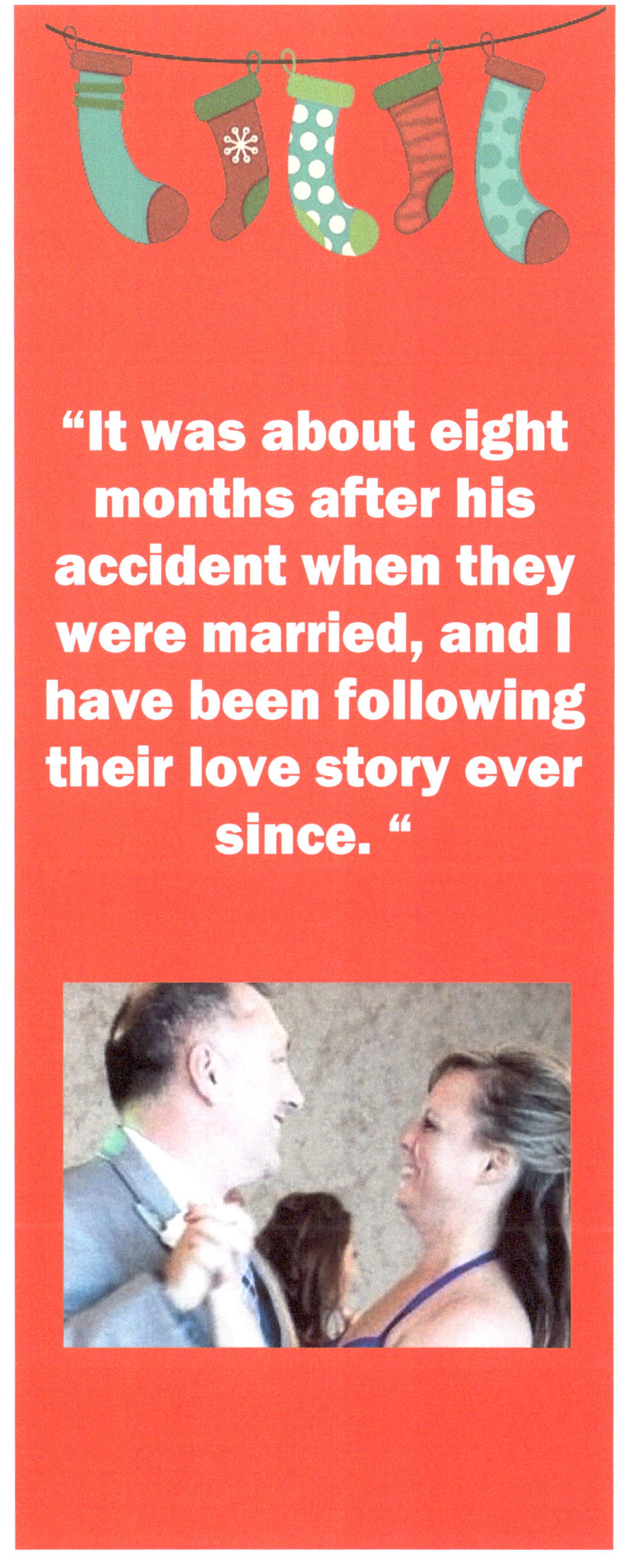

Every year Paul and Tammy testify before the Department of Safety and Homeland Security in an effort to change the helmet laws in their state. The bill has been tabled each year, but they continue to press ahead.

This year Paul met an incredible goal of returning to the work force. Paul in his own right is an incredible human being, but when the fight inside of him is partnered with the determination inside of his wife, Tammy, they are truly amazing! This is what love can do…it can take us further than we ever dreamed, despite incredible obstacles.

Meet Nicole Bingaman

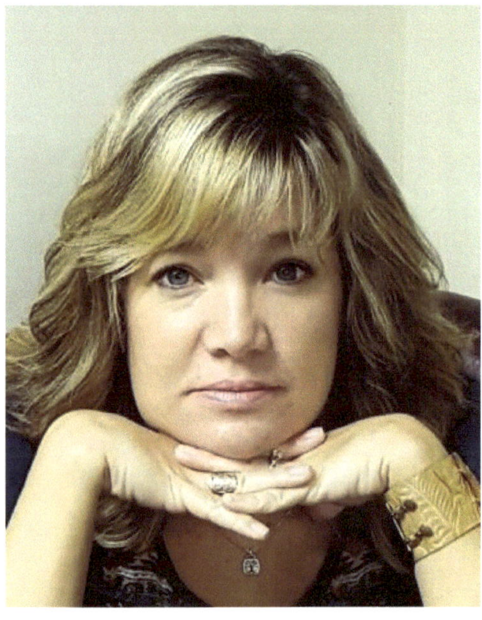

Nicole has worked in the human service field for over twenty years. Since Taylor's injury Nicole has become an advocate and spokesperson within the TBI community.

Nicole's book "Falling Away From You" was published and released in 2015. Nicole continues to share Taylor's journey on Facebook. Nicole firmly believes in the mantra that "Love Wins."

Pretty No More

*What will you do when I'm
Pretty no more?
When my arms don't work,
And I can't hold the door?
When my mind is too slow,
Yet it won't take a break,
So clamoring racket is all
My mouth makes.*

*What will you do when I
Forget all I've learned?
And I stumble while watching
Old relationships burn?
What will you do when I drool
While I smile?
And when it takes me two hours,
To walk just a mile?*

*Will you stop and notice
Who I am now?
Will you vow to be present,
Yet evade me somehow?
Will you pretend not to notice me,
When I'm in the store?
Will your actions declare,
"We are friends no more?"*

*I did not ask for all of the changes you see.
The truth be told, I'd rather be free.*

*Who I am now I must strive
To accept.
This new version of me is all
I have left.
What will you do when I'm
Pretty no more?*

Finding Senior Housing can be complex, but it doesn't have to be.

Call A Place for Mom. Our Advisors are trusted, local experts who can help you understand your options. Since 2000, we've helped over one million families find senior living solutions that meet their unique needs.

"You can trust **A Place for Mom** to help you."

– Joan Lunden

a Place *for* Mom.

A Free Service for Families.

Call: (844) 578-9504

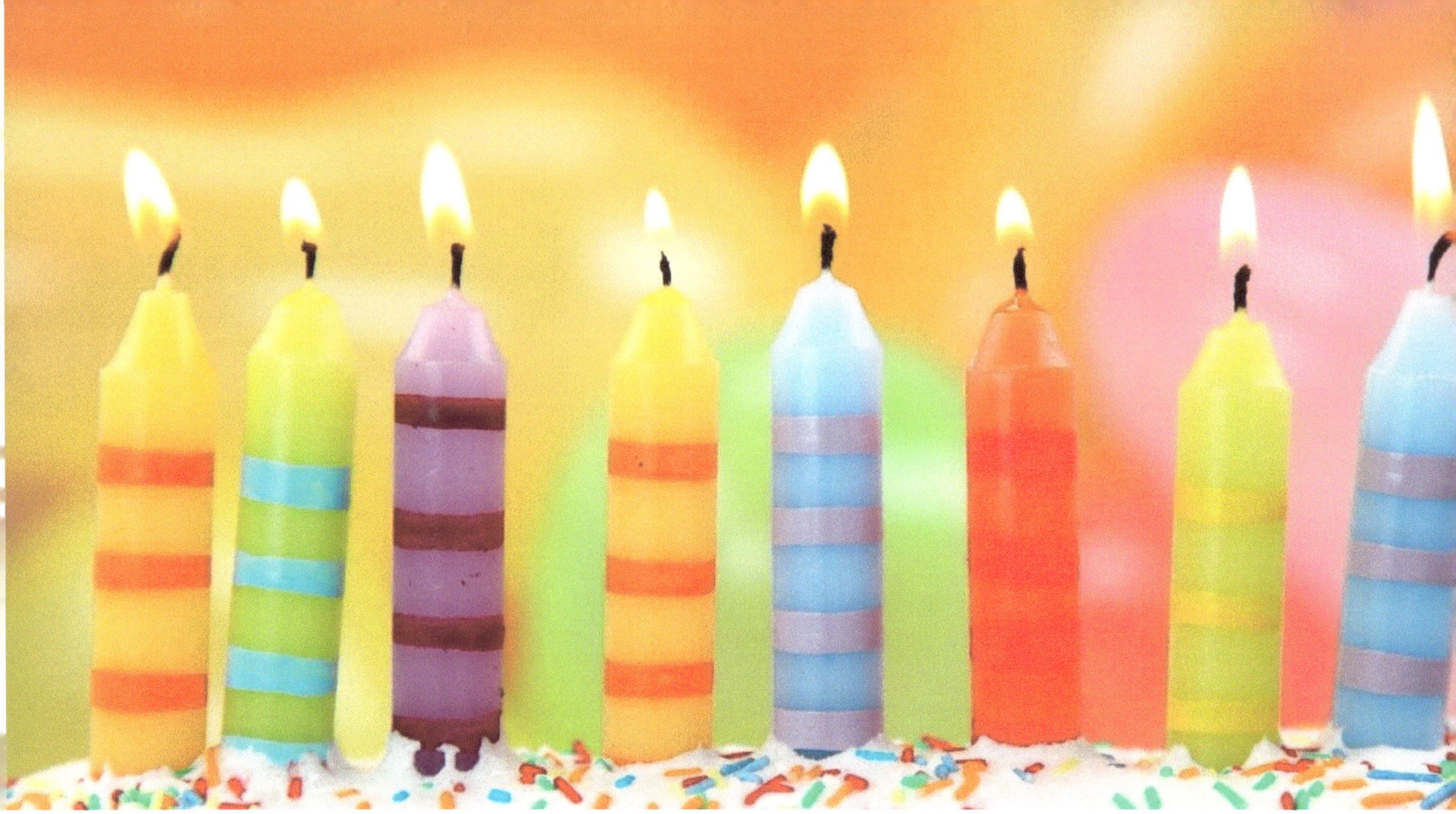

Turning Fifty

By Michelle Bartlett

This year I turn fifty years old. It is a big accomplishment for me. On Canada's 100th birthday, I was born in a small town in St. Stephen, New Brunswick. So on Canada's sesquicentennial, the year has been full of celebration across the country. Many of the same traditions from the centennial celebrations were included in this year's celebrations. The Canadian Mint circulated special commemorative currency, and many spectacular events have been held coast to coast.

My journey into the "brain injury community" began innocently. At the age of thirty-six, I met the man of my dreams. We wanted to start a family but, I had a history of heart disease. We had been told by the doctors that in order for me to carry a healthy baby to full-term, I would need surgery to have my heart repaired. We were told about the risk of complications and we did not even give it a second thought. I wanted to have a healthy life, a healthy baby, and a healthy marriage with my future husband.

Just prior to my surgery, my father passed away after a lengthy illness. We had already talked about the surgery and my upcoming marriage. He approved of both. I was grateful to have his blessing. That is a comfort to me now. Shortly after my Dad passed away, the hospital called me. There had been a cancellation for the first week of March and they asked if I wanted it. I said yes. The pre-op was done and surgery was scheduled shortly after.

My aortic valve was replaced and my mitral valve repaired. My aorta was also widened to allow for proper circulation. It was a bigger operation than the surgeon had first anticipated. It took him over nine hours to complete, instead of the three hours that he had planned.

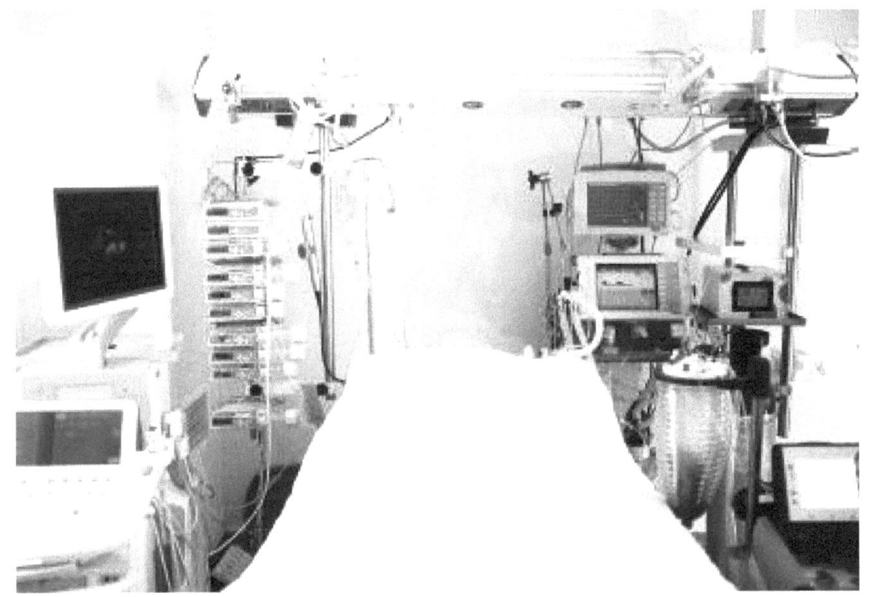

The surgery was deemed a success. I was moved from Intensive Care to the Step-Down Unit within days. On my second day in the Step-Down Unit, I went into cardiac arrest. My lungs and heart had completely stopped. The doctors and nurse estimate I was without any oxygen to my brain for five to seven minutes. It took them hours to stabilize me enough to transfer me to ICU.

MRI and CAT scans were run to check on brain function. There was none. My diagnosis was brain dead with virtually no hope of recovery. The doctors still had me on life support, waiting for my family to make the decision that no family should have to make about their loved one. Three days later, they pulled me off life support and transferred me to palliative care in another hospital.

Coincidentally, seventy-two hours after arriving in palliative care, my best friend was brushing my long, matted hair with a wire brush and I exclaimed, "OUCH!" My "ouch" moment frightened my friend and it circulated thru the hospital very quickly. It is not a regular occurrence that a palliative care patient, in a deep coma, with a diagnosis of brain dead and no hope of survival, actually talks.

Within hours, I was rushed back to the local trauma center. Once I was admitted, the neurologists scheduled another MRI and CAT SCAN. According to the new tests, they showed that now there was brain activity. Against all odds, I had begun to emerge from the coma! Waking up from a coma isn't like you see on TV. The damsel doesn't magically wake up as soon as Prince Charming gives her a kiss. I only wish it was that easy. Emerging back to the conscious world requires time, lots and lots of time.

My emergence took place over several weeks. Gradually I began to recognize faces and remember names of family and friends. I had to learn how to swallow again, to eat, to go to the washroom, to dress myself, and to walk. I was moved to Rehab once I became stable. There the real work began. I had daily Occupational Therapy, Physical Therapy, and in the beginning, Speech Therapy. I progressed rapidly, so rapidly that I was discharged after only three weeks of in-patient rehab. My outpatient rehab would continue for a year or more.

> ## "My emergence took place over several weeks."

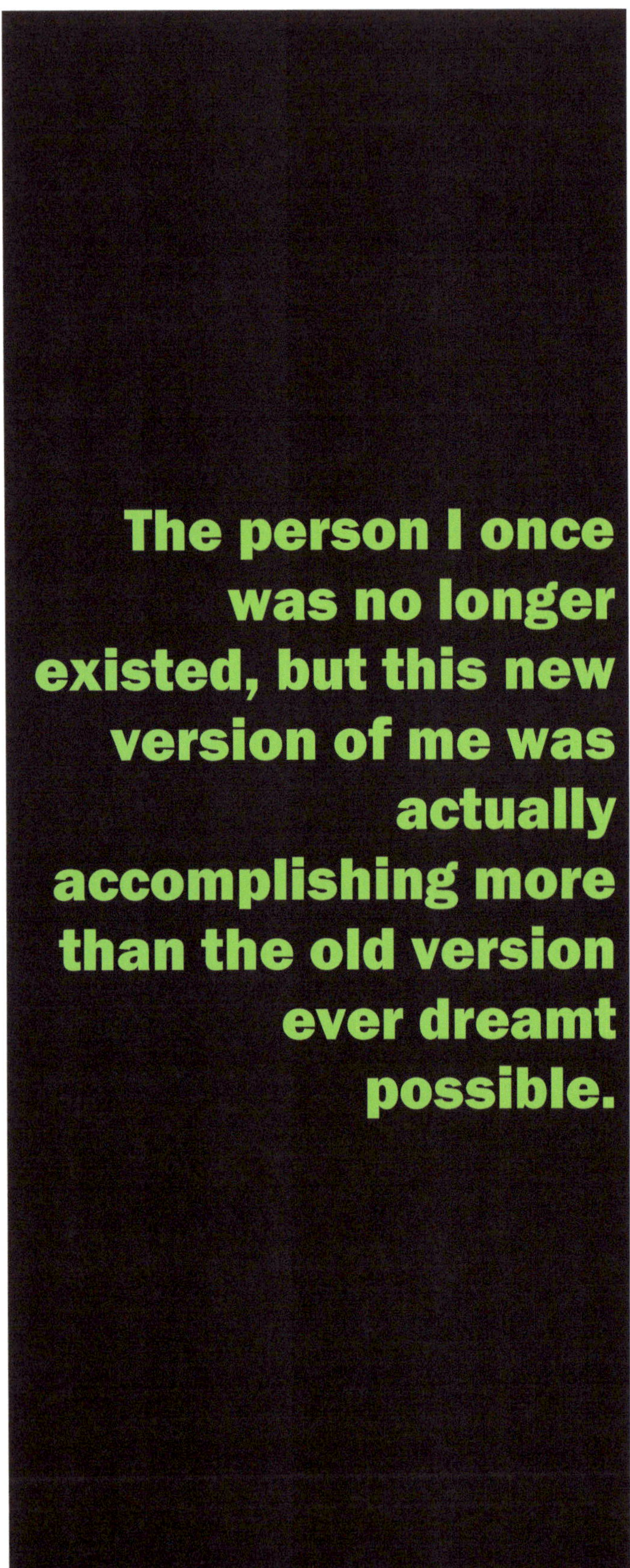

During my rehab, I got married to my fiancé and we got a beautiful cocker spaniel pup we named "Molly." My husband's job required him to be away from home for months at a time. We made the decision to move across the country to be closer to his work. He worked long hours and was away most of the time. Molly and I spent our days in a new, unfamiliar environment looking for a way to fit in.

Within months, I found a group of local Brain Injury Survivors who were just like me. It was a pivotal moment in my life. We had so much in common. It wasn't just about our brain injuries. Our injuries were unique. Each one different, like a snowflake. We shared so many things in common.

The term "neuroplasticity" had just become popular at this time and I remember the excitement in our little group. It gave us the one thing we had all been missing. We now had hope! We had hope that someday, somehow, we could improve. We could read again. How about writing or being independent? Maybe we could even organize a conference. How does public speaking sound? The possibilities were now endless!

My family, especially my mom and husband, immediately noticed the difference in me. They saw the dark cloud of depression slowly lifting. I began getting more involved in the community I lived in. As I did more and more, both my self-confidence and self-esteem soared.

The person I once was no longer existed, but this new version of me was actually accomplishing more than the old version ever dreamt possible. My husband and I separated shortly after my Mom passed away. I had always been told I would never be independent again, but Molly and I moved into an apartment of our own.

After a couple of years of living in my little apartment and Molly and I enjoying our own little family life, I discovered that I needed another heart surgery. The first surgery was extensive and required a long recovery. As I didn't have any support where I was living, I decided to move back across the country to be closer to my family and have the surgery.

I left all of my brain injury supporters. It wasn't easy. As things turned out, I didn't need surgery after all.

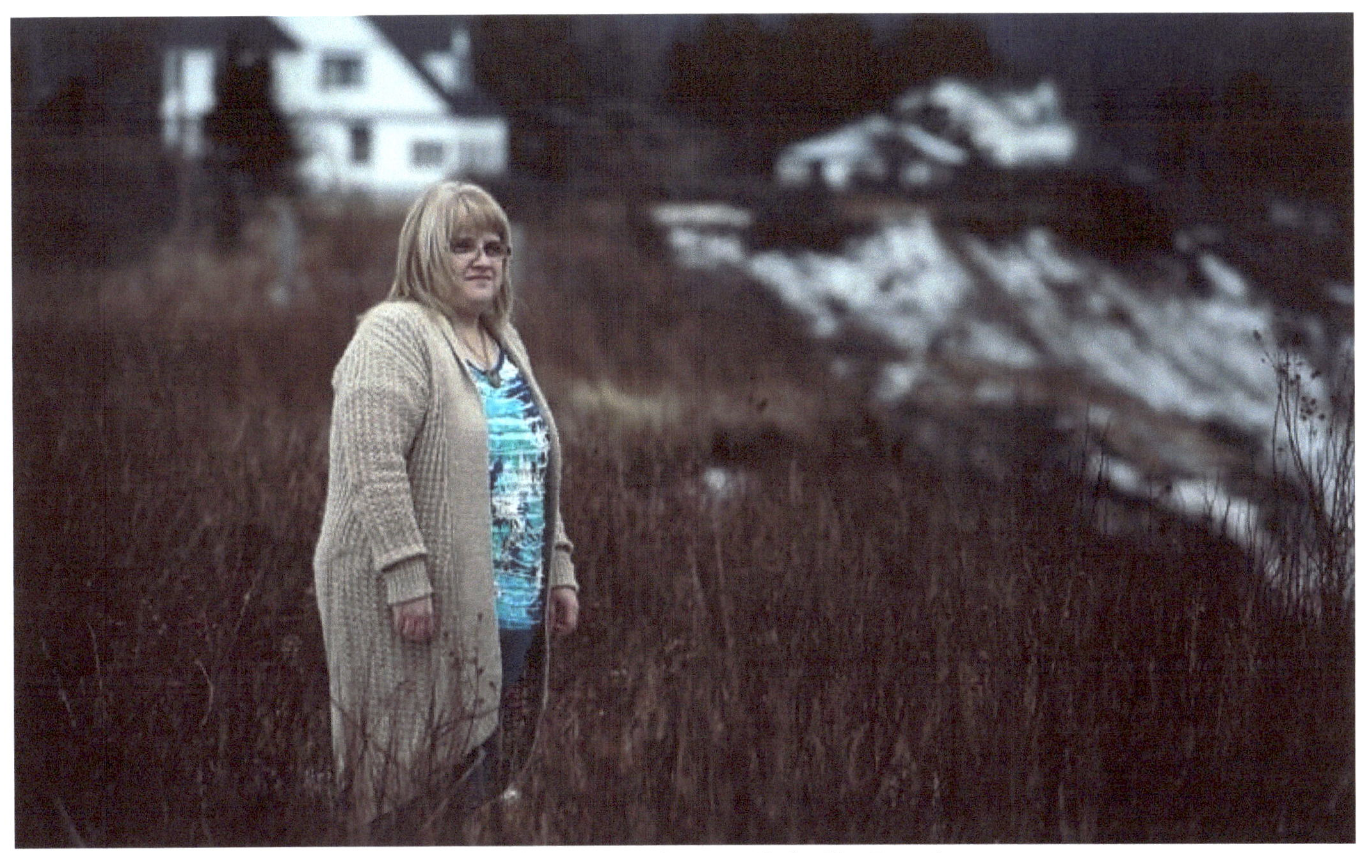

Brain Injury Survivor Michelle Bartlett
Photo Credit: Telegraph Journal

Moving was hard and very complicated. Essentially I picked up and packed up Molly and my life and moved back across the country yet again. I wasn't sure that I was capable of doing it without any support system in place. My brain injury friends came and helped with what they could. Moving day finally arrived and Molly and I were ready to say goodbye to our life and start our new journey.

We took an airplane. Molly was in cargo due to her size. I almost missed my connection by seconds and was close to having a full-blown panic attack. We both arrived safely at our destination, where my family was waiting to greet us.

We settled in to our life again. I am an avid computer geek. I began researching and looking for other brain injury survivors to talk with, share, and support. Helping others helps me cope with my own brain injury. I always say if I have made one person's day brighter, or if my words have been of comfort to them, then my day has been a success.

The last year has been full of many highlights. In 2016, I was one of the keynote presenters at the Annual Brain Injury Canada Conference held in Toronto. I was presented the Award of Merit from Brain Injury Canada. I considered this a huge accomplishment for myself. It was my first time public speaking.

"I was presented the Award of Merit from Brain Injury Canada."

In April 2017, I was the keynote presenter for the Brain Injury Canada Semi-Annual Conference held in my hometown of Saint John, New Brunswick. I was also a member of the conference organizing committee.

Late in the summer, Molly, my beloved cocker spaniel who was now twelve became seriously ill. She was diagnosed with a fatal form of heart disease. Medications would only work short-term. She crossed the rainbow bridge on August 18th. I am still adjusting to life without her. Days are easy now and the nights are improving. Molly kept me strong. She relied on me. She loved me unconditionally.

I still keep in touch with all of the people I have met over the years. I don't see the injury; I see the person's heart, their soul. Turning fifty isn't all that bad. I thought I would never reach it. Here I am now an advocate for other survivors, a new writer, and blogger. I know there is more to find. It's actually kind of exciting. Now I accept the good days along with the bad. There is no ending to my story yet and only I can write it.

Meet Michelle Bartlett

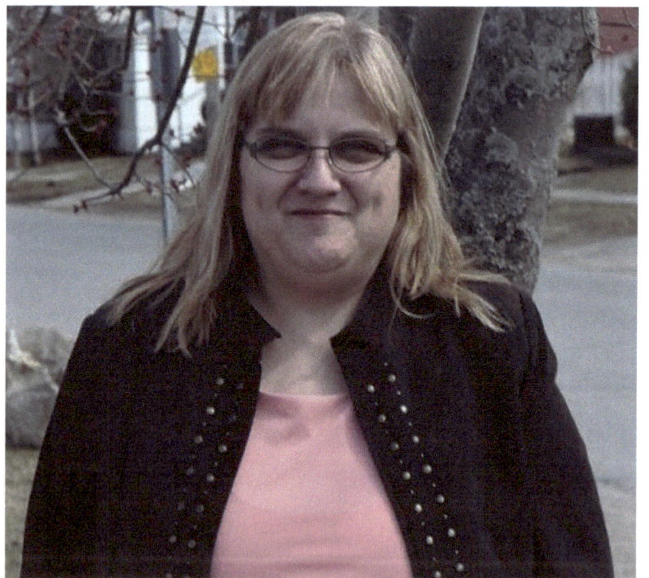

Michelle is a community advocate as well as a facilitator for brain injury survivors and their families and supporters. She suffered a severe anoxic brain injury in 2004 and has become very interested in brain injuries and psychology. She wants to learn and understand, and give back to the community that helped both her and her family during a very difficult time in their lives. She has come a long way from the early days being unable to care for herself and still has a long journey ahead of her. Now as an advocate for Brain Injury Canada, she feels strongly that she has a voice for the people that sometimes feel that their voices cannot be heard.

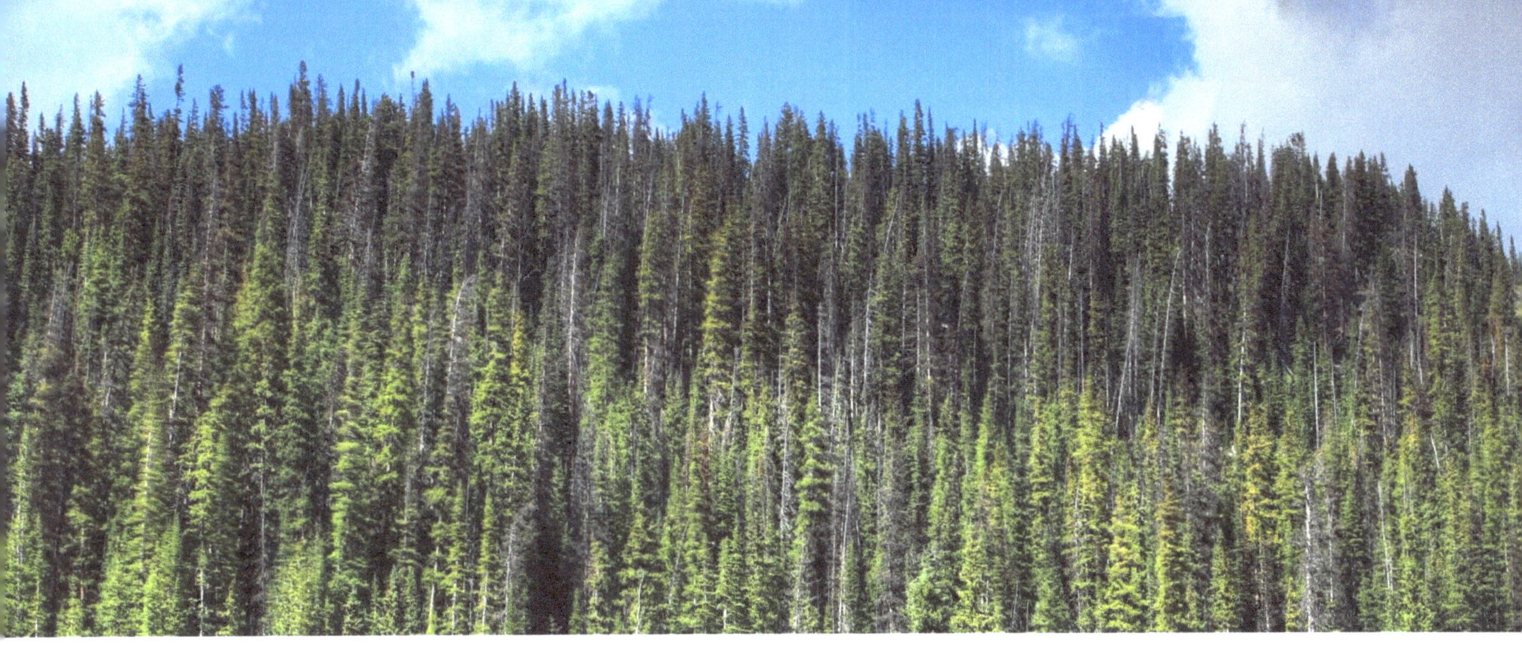

Life Goes On

By Keely Parker

August of 2014 was the worst month of my entire life. On August sixth, after returning from a night out with my mum and sisters we found my dad dead. He had a cardiac arrest while home on his own. Only sixty-nine years old and the most amazing father, he was now unexpectedly gone. We were all devastated. On the sixteenth of August, only ten days after the passing of my dad, I was scheduled to fly to San Francisco with my husband and son and others for a family holiday to visit Yosemite National Park, and then to Las Vegas. My husband and son left on Saturday and I rescheduled my flight until after my dad's funeral.

I joined my family a few days later in Pine Mountain Lake. This is a beautiful place for reflection and gave me time to digest what had happened. We then went on to Vegas. Since we got married in Vegas, we thought it was fitting to go back for our anniversary. That night my life changed forever. At midnight, after returning from downtown Las Vegas and a lovely anniversary meal, I fell down the stairs of a double decker bus and landed on my head, waking only a few seconds later shouting, "I feel like someone is stamping on my head, I feel like my head is going to explode."

> **"I fell down the stairs of a double decker bus and landed on my head."**

The next few weeks are pretty much a blur for me. After a subdural hematoma, a fractured skull, intensive care and a week in hospital, I was allowed to travel back home to the UK. Back in the UK with limited vision, dizziness, confusion, a neck collar, a walking stick and serious need to sleep all the time, I was starting to try to make sense of where I was. I had not required surgery, I had not broken anything,

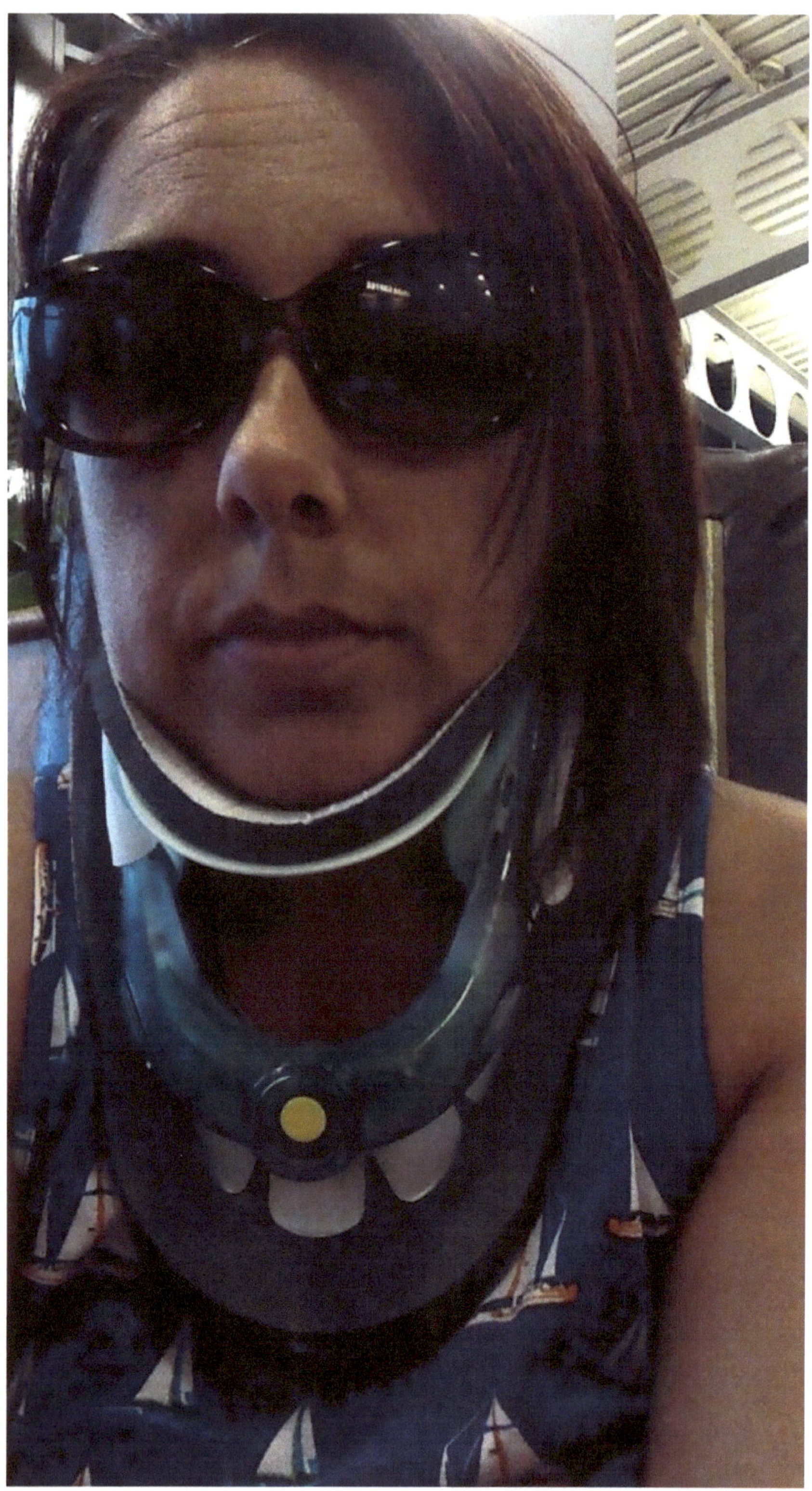

yet I was still struggling to walk due to balance problems and ongoing dizziness. I couldn't drive, due to my fractured skull. I was unable to see because I had blood in my eyes.

Everything was so confusing. The next few months were full of hospital appointments and sleep. I remember telling one specialist that I would be back at work in October, even though I still could not walk properly, drive, or even follow a conversation for more than a few minutes without forgetting something or getting confused.

I was/am a teacher and have always been very proud of that fact. It was at some point during this time that I realised I had no taste or smell. Turns out, I had also sheared my olfactory nerve.

Thankfully, things did get easier than those first few months. My balance improved. Though not as it was before, it was better. I no longer walk with a stick and only have balance problems when fatigued. My eyesight improved months later when the blood dispersed. The neck improved so the collar disappeared.

The biggest challenge for me is the fatigue. This has massively reshaped my new life. I have to manage everything in order to be able to function in a way that I am happy. I eventually tried to return to my old job but it just took too much out of me. In the UK, teachers work till 11:00 PM doing tasks like marking and planning. I wasn't able to do that any longer. I could not manage a normal 9 to 5 day, never mind teacher hours. The self-doubt and the negativity is also hard for me to cope with but I am managing it.

Since I have stopped trying to get back to the old me and started to embrace the new me, I am so much happier. The old me was very ambitious and hardworking. The new me likes to do a good job, but also likes time to relax. These days, I take long walks with my dog and breathe in the fresh air. The old me never got stressed about little things, but the new me gets anxious about lots of things. I have to plan and strategize to try to minimise this. The old me said "yes" to everything, while the new me knows that I have limitations and that it's okay to say no if I need to. The old me took many things for granted. The new me notices the sunrise, the sunset, and the way the trees move in the breeze. The new me really sees more beauty in the world than she ever saw before.

A TBI is never something I would have chosen. My life is very different now, but not all of it is bad. Three years on and I have lots of things to be thankful for. I have a husband who stuck by me and I am a successful home tutor, now working for a few hours a day. I even started back yoga this week. Life does indeed go on.

Meet Keely Parker

Born in Nottingham in the UK, Keely is the middle child of three girls. She was ill as a child with ulcerative colitis and had a colostomy for six months but this healed and from the age of ten, she enjoyed her childhood. She had a loving hardworking mum and dad. She loved school, loved her friends, her sisters and going to drama club.

She is currently a home tutor working with students who can't cope with school for various reasons and she also does private tutoring for students in sociology. She now lives with her very supportive husband, a PE teacher and her twenty-four year old son and her healing dog, Chase.

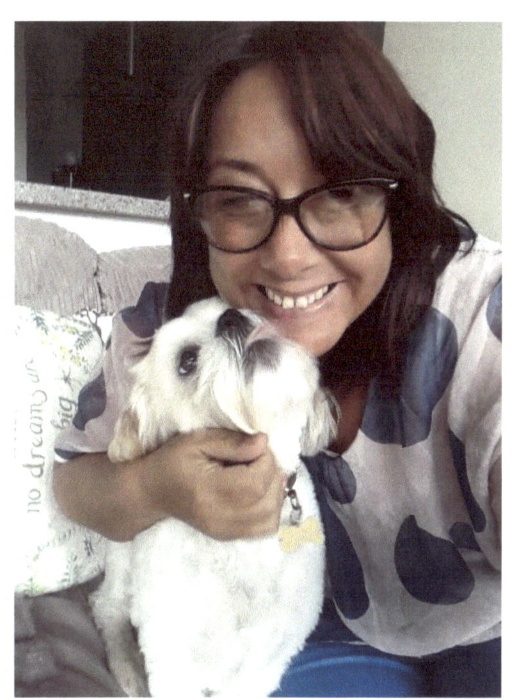

Join our Facebook Family

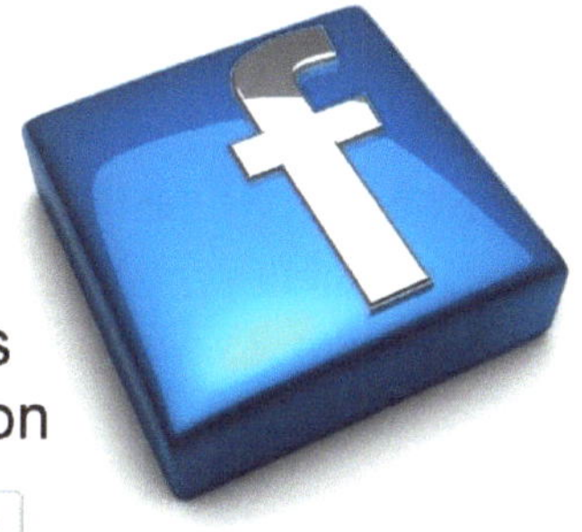

What do over 25,000 people from over 40 countries and five continents all have in common? They are all members of our vibrant Facebook family at /TBIHopeandInspiration

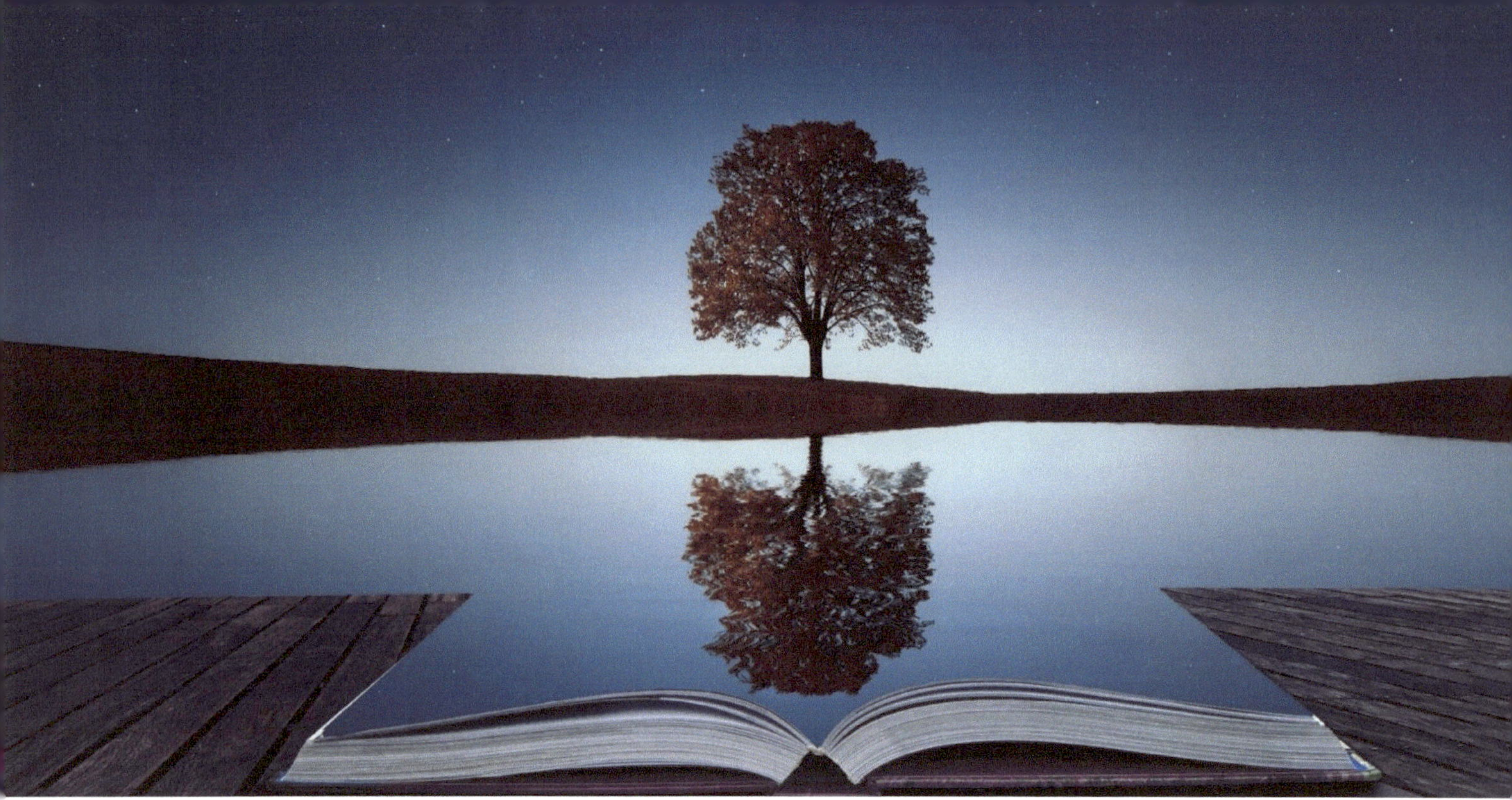

Reflections on Life after Brain Injury
By Hilary Zayed

Why is it that our reflection in the mirror is not what others see? I see a little less color, an imperfect smile, and a drabby look, while others see me as colorful, beautiful and full of life. I hear it all the time, "You look great!"

I cannot open my head to reveal the injured tissue inside my skull that makes my life unrecognizable to me. I look at myself and see someone incapable of safely taking care of herself. Unable to independently support myself, unsure of what I can and cannot do, shaking and crying, the pots and pans banging inside my brain, I fall limp with my vision closing in. My refracted, deflected image to the outside world is not my true reflection. Most of the time I am okay with "You look great," as I hear the un-uttered words, "for someone who says they have so many problems."

I have a choice. I can reflect "thank you," or I can refract. "You only get to see me when I am well enough to be out and about."

> **"I cannot open my head to reveal the injured tissue inside my skull that makes my life unrecognizable to me."**

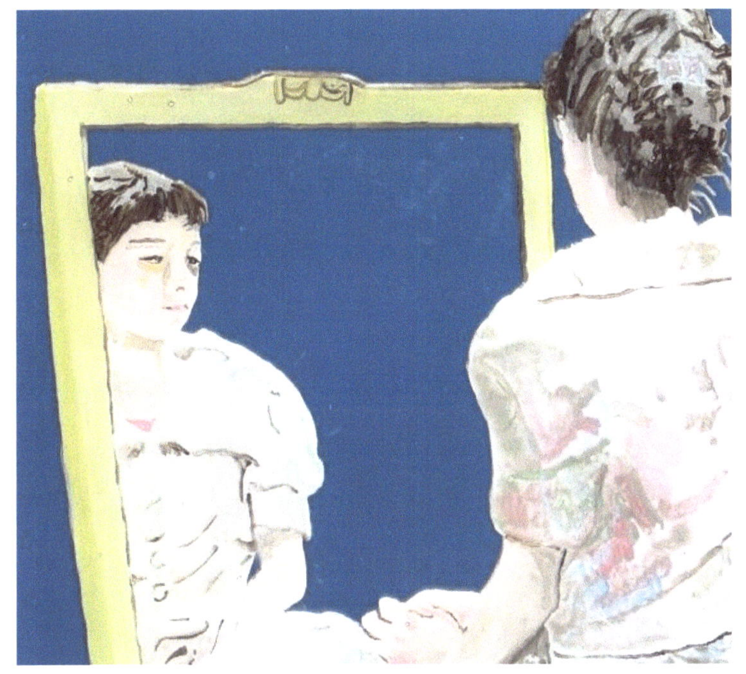

This picture shows a girl looking into the mirror. She sees something different than what other people are telling her they see. Often as a person with a hidden disability there comes the decision of how much to reveal to the disbeliever. I thought my role was to educate others about my traumatic brain injury and recognize that what they thought about that was their decision.

I still find myself in that situation as I now see myself as an advocator for those with brain injuries. However, to get to that point I had to explore my own feelings about my hidden disabilities, decide how much to share, and how to deal with their response. What I learned was that the outcome could fall within the range of not being invited along with a person because they might be afraid of what they don't understand, to the other side of the spectrum where they understand and bring you along offering support. Either way, I have learned that I know my needs and my truth and that leads me to take better care of myself and advocate and educate without fear.

Has anyone ever said to you, "You look great!?" The challenges of living with a hidden disability make me feel that I have often been told that I don't seem disabled or that I look "fine." This makes me feel as though I have to explain how hard it is to live with a brain injury and that they don't believe me. I have had to learn that it is the other persons' perception, not mine. I can attempt to educate them and know that I need to advocate for myself as I know my truth. I now have an affirmation that I am fond of… *"I know myself, my needs, and my truth."*

Meet Hilary Zayed

Hilary Zayed reinvented herself as an artist, writer, educator and speaker of the TBI experience after falling from her horse in 2006. As an active member of Brain Injury Voices in Portland, Maine, she devotes her capable volunteering time to sharing her TBI experience by educating, advocating and supporting others in the brain injury community. Her book, Reinventing Oneself After Loss, An Artful Insight published by Lash Publishing, and her website www.reinventingoneself.com were developed to share her experience of moving forward through art and writings.

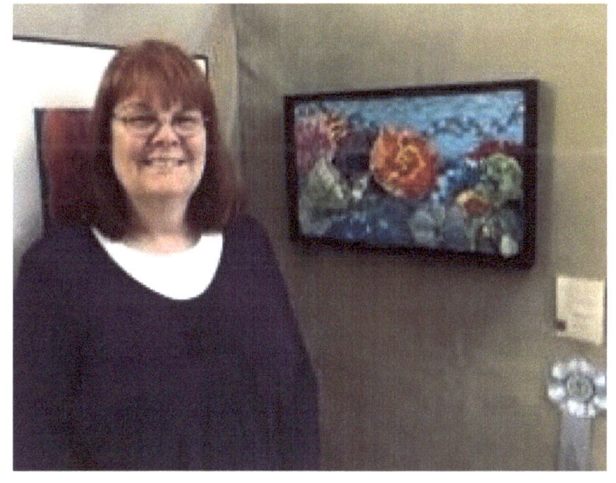

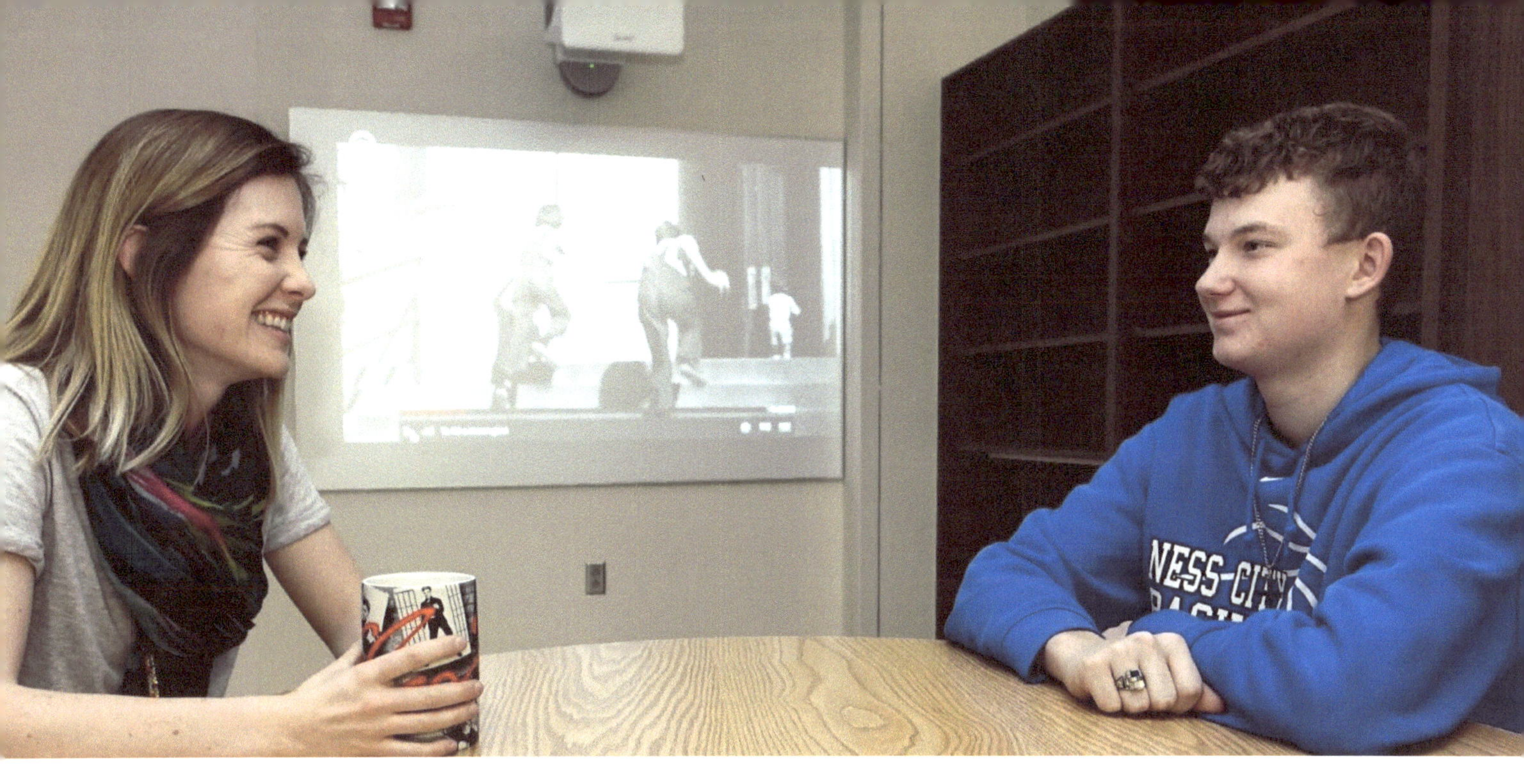

Dayton Copeland – A Success Story

Submitted By Marjorie Sturgeon, Madonna Rehabilitation Hospitals

"It's been awhile. How are you doing?" asks a former nurse.

Dayton Copeland receives a warm welcome from the pediatric care team at Madonna's Omaha Campus. "Just kind of excited to see everyone again and here for a different reason," said Dayton.

The Kansas teen is here today to reunite and catch up with his former nurses and therapists on what he's been up to over the summer.

"Umpiring baseball games, playing basketball," he said.

Dayton is heading back to school in the fall after suffering a traumatic brain injury in December 2016 stemming from a two-vehicle car crash near his home in Ness City, Kansas. "[Dayton] came to us not speaking, not opening his eyes, not looking up. He could sit in a wheelchair partially, with some help and not really responding to outside stimulus much," said Dr. Sheilah Snyder, a Madonna Rehabilitation Hospitals' physician.

In the early days, Dayton's family relied on faith, prayers, and Madonna for hope. "The first day, they came in and said, 'Well, we're going to walk,'" recalls Angela Copeland, Dayton's mom. "Two of them got him up from the wheelchair and they parked him right here. I'm sitting here, going 'what? He's not even awake. How are you going to walk him?' They helped him stand up and one of them held his head, while the other touched his leg and said, 'Take a step, Dayton.'"

Angela says New Year's Eve is when her son seemed to wake up, becoming more aware of his surroundings and situation. Through intense physical, occupational and speech therapy, he made tremendous progress before heading home in March.

"When I got out of here, I started golfing right away," said Dayton.

Now he's gearing up for deer season.

"He loves to hunt, so we've been building blinds and starting to get on to doing mounts," said Nathan Copeland, Dayton's father.

"The amount of therapy that he got as intensely as he got, is absolutely the reason he's recovered as quickly as he has. He was here for quite a long time but he's made extraordinary steps in his recovery. I would not have thought he would be going back to school this year if you would have asked me last winter," said Dr. Snyder.

With the type of brain injury that he had, most people do not come out of it like this and he's almost his old self," said Angela.

 "These people were part of our family for a long time. We miss them but we didn't want to be there in that situation again. They'll always have a place in our hearts and minds," said Angela.

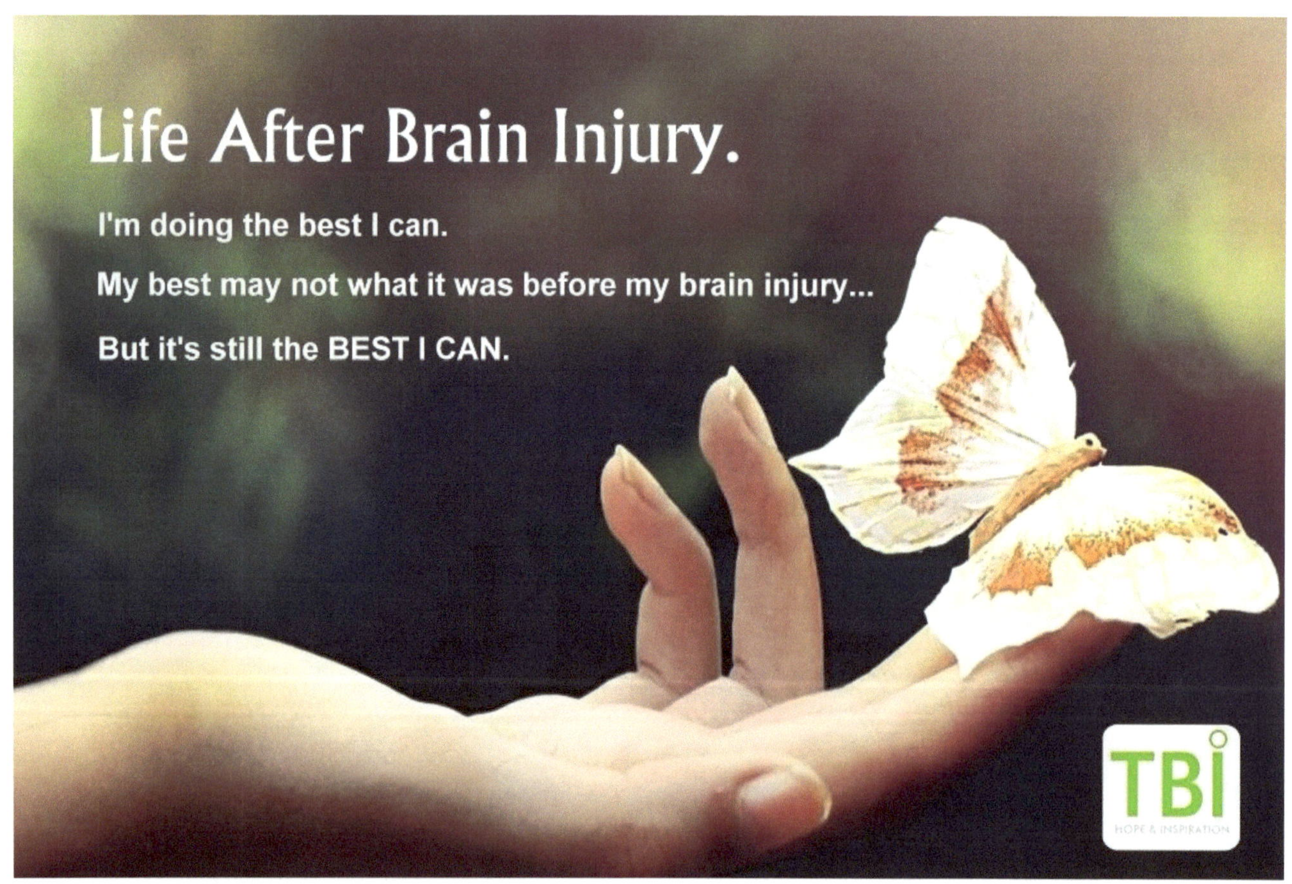

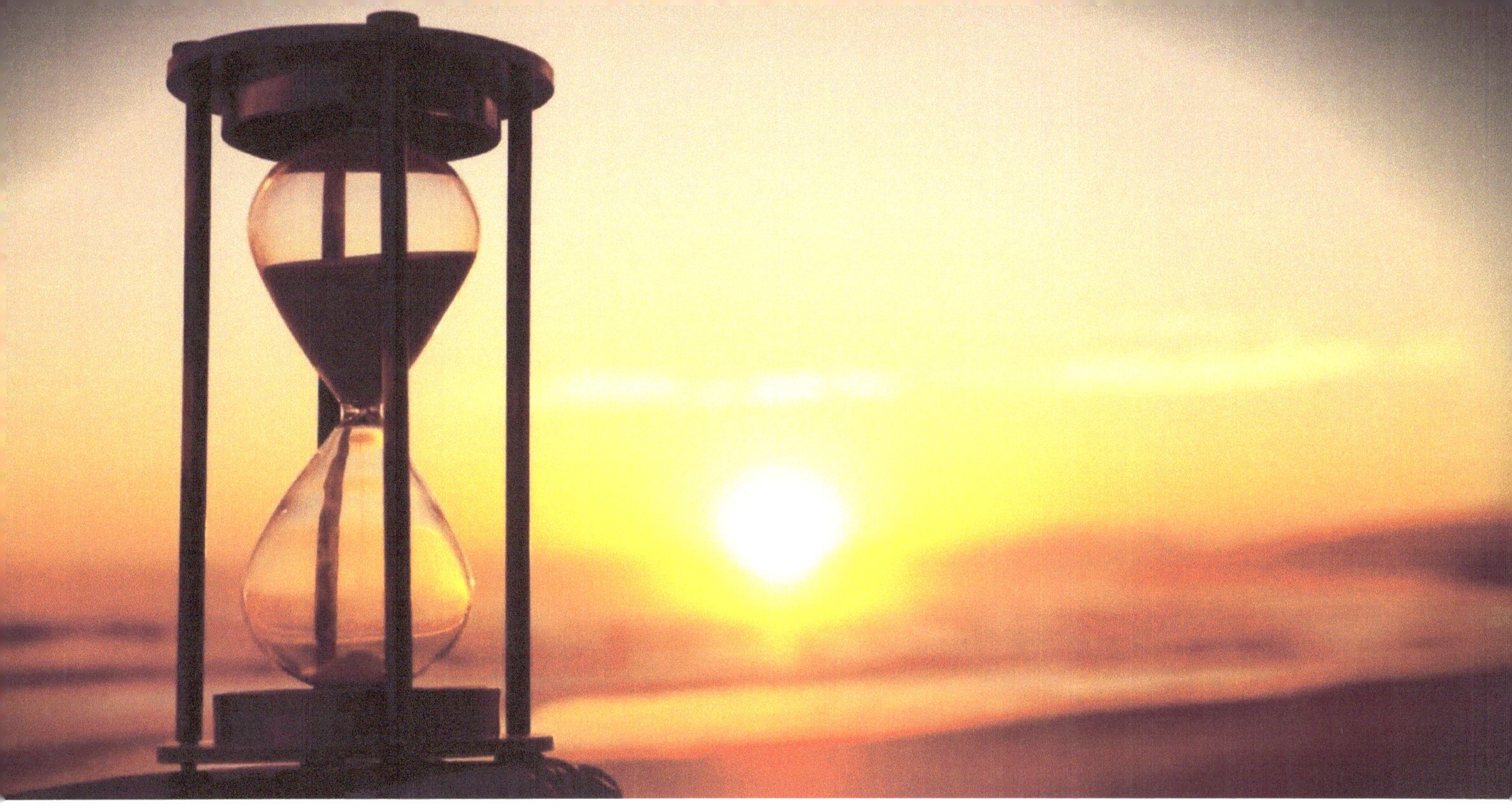

The Power of Yet

By Barbara Stahura

This tiny, common word packs a ton of hope—and your body knows it. "Yet" can be a trusted guide through the Foreboding Forest of Fear or a safe passage across the Ocean of Doubt. It encourages you to keep going when perhaps you would rather just turn around and climb back under the covers. While it does not guarantee success - a fish will never be able to climb a tree, no matter how much it tries - it can improve your odds.

Think of something you want to accomplish but haven't been able to. Maybe it's not as grand as a desire to complete your first marathon, although it can be; perhaps it's just making it around the block after years of too many doughnuts and not enough exercise. Maybe, despite numerous hours of practice with your violin, you still can't play that one passage in "The Lark Ascending" with the right touch of passion, and sometimes not even the right notes. Perhaps your attempts at knitting have several times fallen flat. Or you may be grieving a lost dream and believe you will never be able to release it and move forward.

> **"You may be grieving a lost dream and believe you will never be able to release it and move forward."**

Think about your situation as you sit quietly, eyes closed. Then say aloud several times, "I can't do this," and really mean it. Pay attention to how you feel in your body.

Then do it again, only this time say, "I can't do this—*yet,*" several times with emotion. Once more, pay attention to any physical sensations you might have. Do you feel different than when you said you could not do it? If not, that's fine. But with practice, you will begin to notice that you likely feel lighter and somehow more uplifted. Those sensations are your mind-body at work, instantly transforming your thoughts into the physical sensations that blossom from the hormones and neurochemicals your body produces in response— and building new networks in your brain that will help you reach your goal.

You have just experienced the power of "yet." Can't or can't *yet*: Each one is a story you tell yourself, and each one creates your particular experience of reality.

"Yet" is a marker of a growth mindset that can help you improve your brainpower and motivation over time. In her research with students, Carol Dweck has discovered that, "Just the words 'yet' or 'not yet,' we're finding, give kids greater confidence, give them a path into the future that creates greater persistence.

And we can actually change students' mindsets. In one study, we taught them that every time they push out of their comfort zone to learn something new and difficult, the neurons in their brain can form new, stronger connections, and over time, they can get smarter."

This holds true for you grown-ups too.

You already know the power of journaling, and now you can put the power of "Yet" to work in those pages, too.

Once again, try the experiment above, where you first tell yourself "I can't do this," and then, "I can't do this—yet." After each time, write for a few minutes about the experience: what did you feel in your body? How were your emotions affected? Then compare your writings about the two statements. Which reality would you rather experience?

Another way is to make a brief list of at least five difficult transitions you have experienced over your lifetime, such as a promotion, the birth of a child and the attending exhaustion and fears, heartbreak and grief, illness or recovery, writing your first book. Then for each one, write a few sentences about how at first you were not sure you could navigate the transition and accept the change, and then about how you did. You were experiencing the power of "yet" at those times even if you did not realize it.

You can also use your journal to envision and create your path to the new way. Choose a current transition in your life or one you are considering. Jot down your doubts and fears about moving through to the other side and how you're not sure you can do it. Be honest and open with yourself. Then, write again, but this time, use your imagination to envision the best possible outcome, even if you don't believe it—yet. Over time, you can revise and update this vision as necessary. Writing down your dreams can prove a great help in achieving them.

Meet Barbara Stahura

Barbara is a Certified Journal Facilitator. She has guided people in harnessing the power of therapeutic journaling for healing and well-being since 2007. She facilitates local journaling groups for people with brain injury and for family caregivers at HealthSouth Deaconess in Evansville, Ind., journaling for wellness and well-being classes for Ivy Tech Community College.

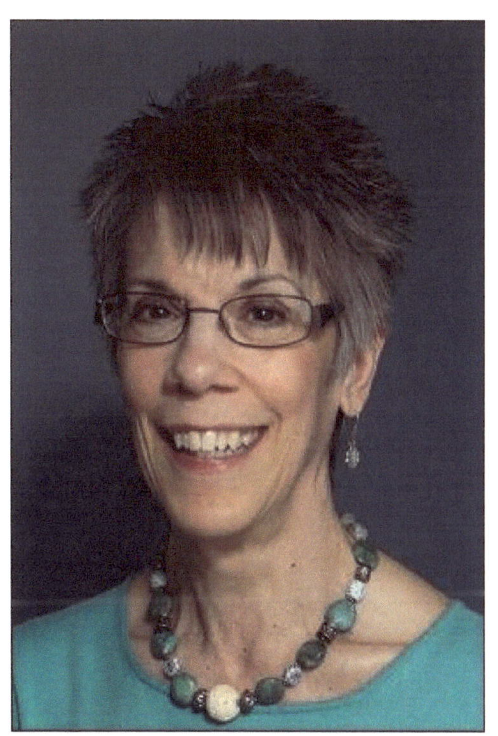

She also presents and has presented journaling events for many statewide Brain Injury Associations/Alliances. Co-author of the After Brain Injury: Telling Your Story, the first journaling book for people with brain injury, she lives in Indiana with her husband, a survivor of brain injury.

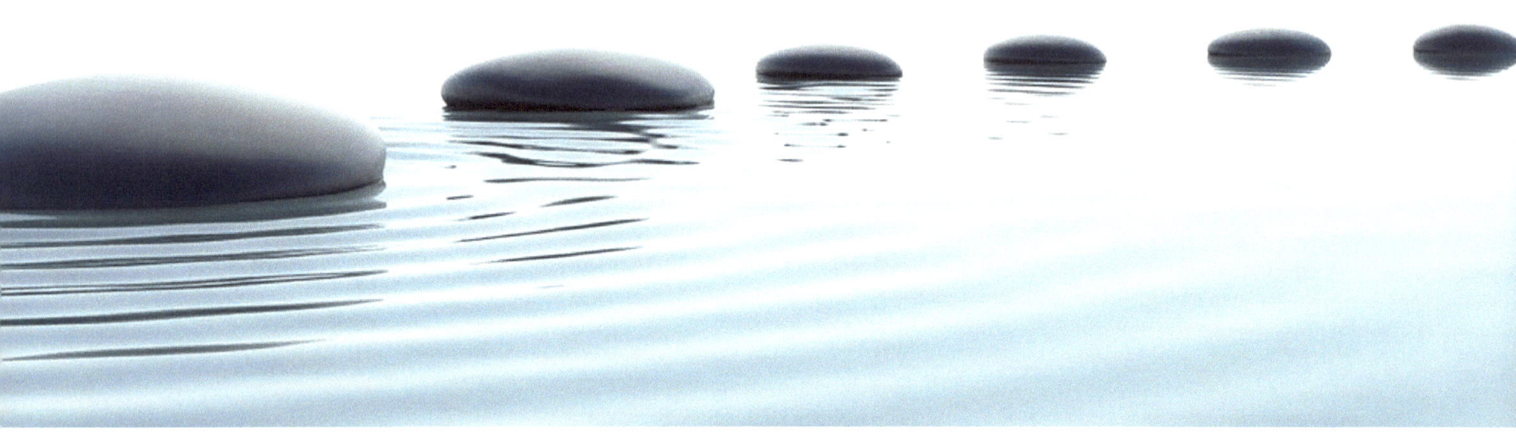

A Simple Life
By Mike Strand

Like everyone says about themselves: before my brain injury, I was above average. I was super smart, athletic, type A, and highly motivated. This also meant that I put a lot of pressure on myself. There was absolutely no reason I shouldn't be a captain of industry, spiritual advisor to the Dalai Lama, and the first president to be elected unanimously.

Of course, those things weren't happening, and as I eased into my mid-twenties I began a gradual descent into despair. I was living a life deferred. I was telling myself that somehow between now and forty this would all happen. I was telling myself everybody would be so shocked when all this happened, even though I knew it would happen all along.

Except that it wasn't happening and, deep down, I knew it never would. I was going to be one of those guys from that Bruce Springsteen song reliving the glory days of my youth. And then something wonderful happened.

> "In one fell swoop, about as big as fell swoops can get, all those hopes and dreams were off the table."

I sustained a severe brain injury.

In one fell swoop, about as big as fell swoops can get, all those hopes and dreams were off the table. It took a gravel hauling semi-truck to knock my dreams away. I almost died, but lucky for me, I tend to live.

Like most people who have suffered an accident like this, I eventually became depressed. I didn't want to live half a life. I didn't want to be in a world with only half the possibilities (and they were the lower half of the range). I raged, I strove, and I willed it otherwise. I made a remarkable recovery, but the best I would ever be is "a very high-functioning person with a brain injury."

My ideas and thoughts, achievements, and surmounted peaks, would always have the brain injury qualifier; i.e., *that was great... for a guy with a brain injury*. I had attained some degree of agency, but without authority. Any argument I made was always suspect. Was I sure? How do you know? The most positive response I could get from any of my assertions was, "Well, I don't know about that…."

So, I wadded up all my ambition and tossed it away. I radically accepted that I was just me, same as everyone else. I wasn't better, smarter, or faster; nor did I have to be. When I truly accepted that, a most wonderful thing happened. This huge onerous weight that I didn't even realize I was carrying, was gone. That was the day I found that I had become a new person. I wasn't trying to be who I would have been if I hadn't had a brain injury. I may not be better, I certainly wasn't worse, but I was most definitely different.

I no longer live a life complicated by ambition. If I want a feeling of accomplishment, I tie my shoes! There was a time when that simple act felt impossible, but that time has passed. I have done things. Hard things. I don't need to prove anything to the world— competition is for other folks. Those poor people who never had brain injuries—they have to continue doing hard things.

I am simply me. I can care and feel, love and be loved, and be immensely happy all the while. I am happy in the here and now.

The hero awakens.

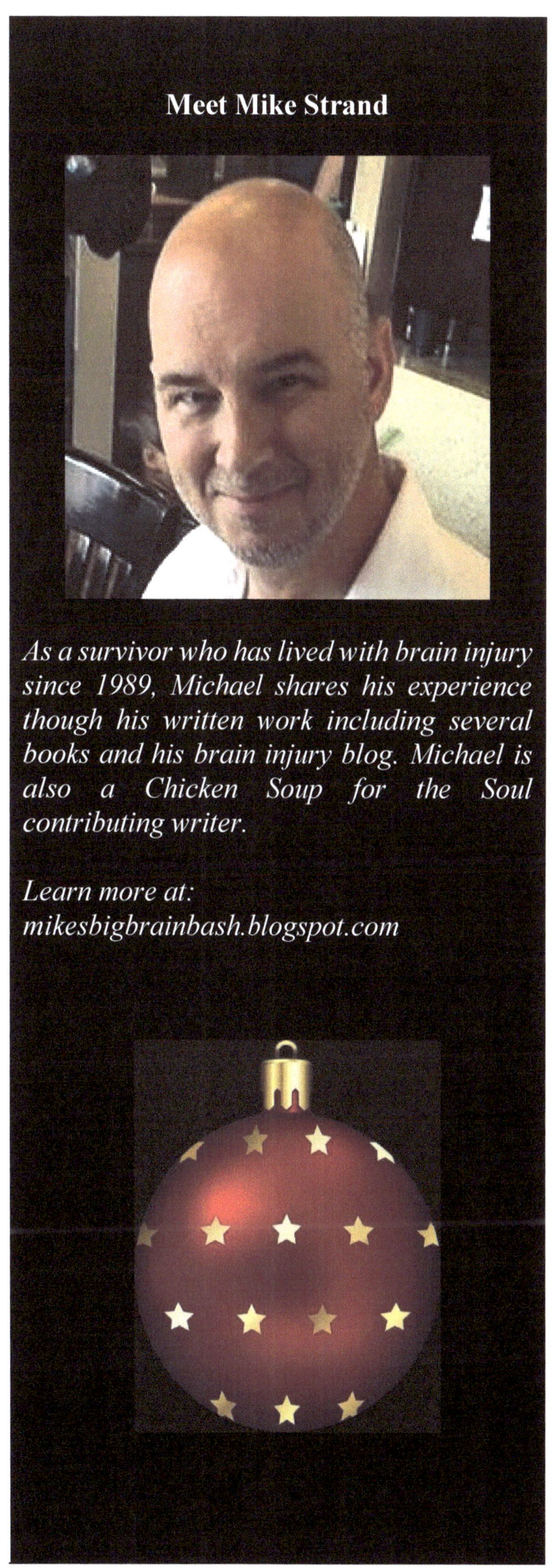

Meet Mike Strand

As a survivor who has lived with brain injury since 1989, Michael shares his experience though his written work including several books and his brain injury blog. Michael is also a Chicken Soup for the Soul contributing writer.

Learn more at:
mikesbigbrainbash.blogspot.com

News & Views

I'm going to let you in on a little secret. A few years ago, I started a new holiday tradition. There were no halls to deck, no bells to jingle, just a new annual tradition that seemed to spontaneously happen one year.

This time of year, the red-kettled Salvation Army volunteers show up at many of the retail locations in our area. This year they were out before the Thanksgiving holiday, something that does not bother me one bit. The Salvation Army maintains relatively low overhead with 82% of every dollar going to aid those they serve.

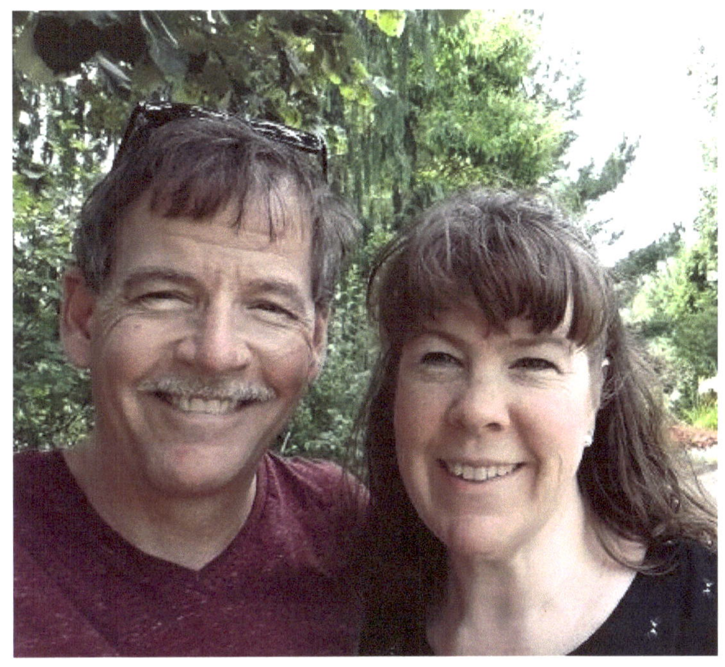

I make it a point to never pass a red kettle without dropping in a dollar or two. I make note of those times that I pass by without a dollar in my pocket and double up at the next passing. It's now been many years since I've not dropped more dollars than times I've passed them by. On the colder days, I regularly ask the bell-ringer if he or she would like a hot coffee or hot chocolate while I'm inside our local market. Most offer a courteous, "No thank you," however on the colder days, most happily accept the offer.

We are in the season of giving. Giving does not need to take on epic proportions, mindful of what is tax deductible. Small acts of kindness and generosity help others and lift humanity higher. A phone call to someone going through a tough time? Ten minutes of your time can lift someone's spirts for a day – or longer. A random dollar stuffed into the red kettle? It might just help buy a holiday meal for someone in need.

There are innumerable ways to give back. Some cost a dollar here or there, while many are gifts you can give freely – like your time. I encourage you to reflect this season on how you might be able to give back – if even just a little. Kindness is catchy. Compassion is love in action.

From Sarah and me, our best wishes for a happy, reasonably healthy holiday season!

~David & Sarah